# It's Time to Curb Your Carbs

## To Save Your Life
## and Keep Your Dignity

## It's Time For A Cure

### (Volume 1)

## Roy Ruins Wheat

Roy Knight Jr

# ACKNOWLEDGMENTS

This would not have been possible without the research and instruction given by Dr David Perlmutter and Dr William Davis and Dr Daniel Amen, Dr Mercola and Dr Donald W. Miller. The British Medical Journal, the New England Journal of Medicine, NIH's PubMed and Wikipedia also played an important part in the construction of this book. I tried to attribute every passage used from those sources.

Credit also goes to James, for without his comments," No one even knows or cares about this", this project probably would have never gotten started and Kimm, who still thinks she needs her carbs. Special thanks to © Wavebreakmedia Ltd | Dreamstime.com - Composite image of stop diabetes and bread photo and istock photo and Free Digital Images.

# FOREWORD

You're probably thinking, how carbohydrates can be as bad as I'm making them out to be. Can carbs kill? As a consumer, you deserve to know the truth. Why nobody has come out with much of the information in this book, prior to now, I don't know. Most, if not all of the studies that are cited within the pages of this book, somehow got shuffled into their respective agency's file box without ever being released to the public. It took the efforts of two doctors, Dr. William Davis and Dr. David Perlmutter, to bring this information to the forefront in their respective books, *Wheat Belly* and *Grain Brain.*

I'd already decided to quit eating bread when I came across Dr Davis' book Wheat Belly. So it was no surprise to me what I was reading. It just confirmed everything that I was already experiencing. Because of my history of brain damage, my interests lie in trying to regain that which I had lost 31 years ago when I suffered the brain injury. I was hoping to bring back some of the intelligence that I had prior. I just began to realize that I could actually do that two years ago. That is what led me to *Grain Brain* by Dr Perlmutter.

To him I dedicate this book. I would never have been able to accomplish this task if I hadn't followed his recommendations in *Grain Brain.*

I started writing this book for my mother when I published my website, Curb Your Carbs. My mother is fighting cancer for the third time. Both my sisters are diabetic and I was on my way to being diabetic. My father was borderline diabetic for a number of years. This is all because we've always eaten bread, pasta, cereal, pastries and every other grain food we could find. We thought we were supposed to. Weren't grains at the bottom of the food pyramid?

All my life I've been eating this food, which I thought was supposed to be good for me. Ironically this food, that was supposed to be so good for me, is actually worse than most anything I can put in my mouth to eat. It turns out that it's this food that's killing America today. And that's not to mention what it's doing to the rest of the world. It's slowly killing everyone who eats it.

I didn't realize this until I gave it up. Like Dr. Davis, I just decided to give up bread, about 28 months ago. When I did, magic happened. So I gave up all grains. More magic happened. So I gave up all carbohydrates. That was when the most magic happened.

That's when I started to regain some of the losses I experienced 31 years ago when a drunk driver ran a red light and struck the car I was riding in, putting me in a coma for the next month. It wasn't until a month later that they released me from St. Joseph's hospital in Phoenix. Since I'd had a massive stroke while in the coma, I woke up with half of my body paralyzed, which I still live with today.

Living with neurological damage has taught me how to overcome deficits that I thought I would never have to. My paralysis still exists. Even though I'm not fully paralyzed and it's only on my right side that I have deficits, I still have them and they still restrict my abilities immensely. *"About me, how hard it is For me to appear normal"* and *"Weight loss, thoughts from my own journey"* will give you a better idea of what I've had to go through, and what I still live with, to this day. I had thought until last year that the brain loss I sustained could not have been restored. I thought it was lost and gone forever.

While there are ongoing neurological deficits that I still have to live with, my newly found ability to grow new brain cells has been nothing short of miraculous. This is evidenced by my abilities to write this book. Within a four month period, I completed all the articles for this book when I wrote them as posts for the website. To me, that is an astounding feat, especially after needing five days at 12-16 hours a day, to explain my medical condition to my doctors, in a three page statement, *About Me. How hard it is for me to appear normal,* that I wrote, last year. (It took me 30 minutes to complete the first paragraph.)

The only way I could have done this is through the knowledge I gained from Dr Perlmutter's book *Grain Brain*. Article 18 *"Weight Loss, Thoughts from My Own Journey"* will give you an idea of my transformation and what I still have to live with, today. I have been updating it ever since I first started it 28 months ago.

I've learned that while the ADA wants us to watch our intake of fat, it's actually glucose that we should be wary of. It's glucose that gums up your whole system. Sugar does the same thing to a car. If you put sugar in the gas tank, it'll ruin the engine. This is because it gums up everything inside the engine, eventually locking everything up, making it seize. Guess what? Glucose does the same thing in your body, it gums everything up. Sugar breaks down into glucose that floats around in your blood, until it can find some insulin to help it get into your cells to get metabolized. Glucose is as deadly to your body as nicotine, or heroin. The only difference is, it's legal and promoted. This makes me wonder where the ADA was, when the studies that showed all this damage, came out.

Sugar = glucose. Carbs = glucose. Keep that in mind as you read through each article. Whenever I use the term *carbs*, I'm usually referring to bread, cereal and pasta. I'm talking about what makes glucose, in your blood, your body's biggest enemy. It's important to pay attention to the glycemic index whenever you're eating carbs. That will give you a good indication how much, of what you're eating, is going to gum up your works. The higher the food is on the index, the more it will gum up your system.

To keep your system running clean and efficiently, I've learned you need to feed it fuel it likes to use. I've learned by eating a high fat, high protein, adequate fiber, diet, it will set your brain up for optimum growth. I've also learned that you achieve the optimum results without any glucose in your system.

Fat can't gum anything up, unless it's fat that's made by your body. There's only one thing that can make fat in your body, and that is the combination of glucose and insulin. And it's this fat that gums things up, because of what the fat was made from, glucose. You've eaten carbs to create the glucose that created this fat. This fat is what I call dirty fat. It's unhealthier than any fat you can eat.

Fat is not the problem. Cholesterol is not the problem. Your body loves fat. Your body uses cholesterol. Your body can't operate properly without it. Your body would rather have you feed it fat because that's what it burns for fuel. Glucose, on the other hand, can't burn as a fuel. It gets turned into fat by your body so it can burn it for fuel. And that's just the start of the problem with carbs.

As a pre-historic creature, our species subsisted mostly on what we could hunt down to eat, fats and proteins from the game that we were able to catch and kill. When our paleo ancestors couldn't find anything to kill, evolution gave our bodies the ability to digest carbohydrates, so we could eat plants, until we could find more game to eat. Then, when our ancestors learned they could grow their food and started eating from what they could grow from the ground, all these problems started to set in. We traded a danger of not having food, for a hidden danger of the food, we ate, slowly damaging our physiology to the point beyond any repair. This could be blamed on the addiction factor of carbohydrates.

This is what paleontologists call, diseases of our modern lifestyle. What they are, in all actuality, are diseases of carbolism, the addiction to carbohydrates. I know. I used to be a carboholic. I was addicted in the worst way and I live with the consequences, still, today. (Arthritis)

Unfortunately, evolution hasn't given all races in our species time to adapt to the carbohydrate intrusion to our digestive processes, especially for the immense amounts that most people feed their bodies, these days. This is why obesity exists more in races who haven't been away from hunting and gathering for as long as other races like Caucasians. Caucasians have been farming a lot longer than African Americans and longer than Native Americans, who express the weight gain, more so, than most Caucasians. Caucasians started farming over 10,000 years ago. Native Americans have only been farming for a few thousand years.

African Americans were hunter gatherers up until 400-500 hundred years ago, when they were forced to consume a western European diet after being brought over to the Americas as slaves. Native Americans had to make a forced switch to a western European diet after the white man took away their territory. These changes in diet for these two races condemned them to lives of obesity and diabetes, simply because their physiology hasn't had the time to adjust to the carbohydrate diet that Caucasians have been on, since we've been growing this food for 10,000+ years. Those 10,000 years gave Caucasians the ability to adapt their physiology to be able to handle the carbohydrate intrusion a little better than Africans or Native Americans. (About 10% of our population express little to no distress from eating wheat and grains, and it only happens in Caucasians.)

This was until about 30 years ago, when GMO crops made their debut. This new *"wonder crop"* that could now feed more people, but at the cost of nutrition, was making all those, who ate this new wheat, gain weight on an unprecedented scale. Thus, the obesity problem that we live with now. This obesity pandemic is leading into a much bigger problem with pandemics of diabetes, dementia, cancer, heart disease, gastrointestinal disorders, and a multitude of other disorders and diseases. Carbs are the true junk food. It really doesn't get much junkier than this.

It is my contention, that if you remove just one factor out of the equation of any of these diseases, the disease would not exist. The one factor that influences more illness and disease than anything else is carbohydrates and the reason for this book. I feel, it's time for a cure and the most efficient and healthiest manor in which we can reach this cure, is to give up the things which cause all the problems, starchy carbohydrates.

I know what the problem is, too. I hear the comments all the time - "What do you eat, then? What do you expect me to eat?" These are things I hear all the time. "You *have* to have *some* carbs", is the one I hear the most. When I hear that, I hear addiction talking. Addiction is the only reason that we haven't woken up to the facts of what this staple has been doing to everyone who eats it. The addiction of someone's brain, telling them, that this food is too important of a food source to do this much damage. How could something so important to our society, possibly cause, so much damage?

Our food industry has found a way to infiltrate industrial strength glue into our diets and it's had a disastrous effect on the publics' health. It's made a society of glucose addicts, worried about where they're going to get there next fix. It displays itself in thoughts like, what kind of sandwich sound good? Or I'll just get me a quick hot dog, thinking the hot dog is going to be, at least, semi nutritious and it would be, if you took away the bun. When people think hot dog, hamburger, or any kind of sandwich....that in itself, is addiction thinking. Even though you're thinking about the meat inside the sandwich, you're actually thinking about the taste of the whole sandwich, which includes the bread that holds the meat and what other goodies you like to put on your sandwiches. That bread or bun is the part of the sandwich that is addictive. That's the taste that keeps pulling you back to keep putting this food into your mouth to eat. You can't help it. Part II covers how to break that hold, which is important if our society is to kick this horrendous addiction. It tells you why the addiction is so hard to bread, and how to fight the addiction. Part III also covers the benefits of living without the intrusion of a carbohydrates into your body.

My initial weight loss results of giving up bread and the subsequent accomplishments that I've achieved are all due to my new found diet, which over the last two years, has become completely ketogenic (no carbs). I've learned that this is the type of diet that our bodies prefer to digest.

For those who still think "anything in moderation", they're allowing their addictions to speak for them. This is because they don't have full control of their emotions and are listening to their hormones. Unfortunately, all of those who are still addicted (which is roughly 90 - 95% of the population), are listening to their hormones and in turn, condemning themselves to lives of what's found in the first article. Moderation is OK, as far as sunlight is concerned. Moderation of carb ingestion, will still damage your brain, no matter how moderate it is. It'll just take longer for you to see the end results, but they'll be the same. Science doesn't lie and for that reason I'm happy that you're reading this book.

# **<u>WARNING!</u>**

This book provides the warnings that the USDA, the FDA and the ADA or the CDC won't, because of their own addiction to this food, and their association with the food industry

# CONTENTS

iii

Foreword

<u>The Physical Consequences of a Carbohydrate Diet</u>

1.  Carbohydrates, The Newly Found Death Sentence        Pg 01

2   Glucose Addiction; America's Biggest, Worst Addiction    Pg 16

<u>Part II    The Evidence</u>

3   How Carbs Are Responsible For AGEs, Your Ticket To     Pg 22
    Diabetes, Dementia, Alzheimer's Disease, Cancer, Heart
    Disease and More

4   Curbing Carbs For Diabetes Control        Pg 31

5   Carbs and Dementia        Pg 38

6   Carbs and Cancer Go Together Like Beetle and Juice     Pg 46

7   Carbs and High Blood Pressure        Pg 55

8   Carbs and Their Influence in Heart Disease        Pg 63

9   Carbs and Arthritis        Pg 71

10  The Value of Balancing Your Cholesterol        Pg 79

11  The Foundation of LDL Particles        Pg 92

12  Gastric Bypass and the Loss of Ghrelin        Pg 98

13  Where's the Outrage, Where's the Warning        Pg 104

Part III    How To Break The Addiction

14  Carbs How to Cut Back                                    Pg 111

15  Why The Addiction Is So Hard to Break                    Pg 118

16  The Payoff A Life Without Carbs                          Pg124

17  My Life Without Carbs                                    Pg129

18. Weight Loss - Observations From My Own Journey In        Pg137
    Abstaining From Wheat

19  The Glycemic Index Your Guide To Health                  Pg146


20  The Power of Being Thin Lies in Eating Fat               Pg153


21  Where's the Outrage, Where's the Warning                 Pg157


Part IV              Societal Concerns


22  Industry's Concerns of Dispelling Sugar, Wheat,          Pg164
    Corn and Grains From Our Diet

23  Industry's Influence in the Expansion of Carbohydrate    Pg167
    Production

24  The Effects of Carbohydrates On Our Society Throughout   Pg170
    History

25  The Argument For Carbs                                   Pg175

26  Where's The Outrage, Where's The Warnings                Pg177

27  My Thought of Eradicating Carbs From Our Diet            Pg182

Final Thoughts                                               Pg186

Afterthoughts                                                Pg187

About The Author – How hard it is for me to appear no        Pg191

# Part 1


# Physical Consequences of a Carbohydrate Diet

# ARTICLE 1
## CARBS, THE NEWLY FOUND DEATH SENTENCE

I know you've been told that you need your carbs, that they're healthy for you and that whole grains have a lot of fiber. How long were they at the bottom of our food pyramid, when we had one, telling us they should make up the largest portion of our meals? How long have we been heeding this message?

I've been doing it all my life. Haven't you? I've been doing it for as long as they've been selling it to me. Every time I turn on the radio or TV, I'm bombarded with ads for "healthy" fruit drinks, "healthy" high fiber whole grain breads, "healthy" granola, etc, etc, etc. The list goes on and on.

**But what if what you've been told was wrong?**

**What if you don't need them,**

**especially in the quantities you've been told to eat them?**

These are questions that I hear all the time from addicts. How do you expect me to live without them? Don't you have to have some? How else does the body get energy?

Remember the "bet you can't eat just one" commercial? That was Lay's selling us addiction, and we bought it, big time, but we'll get deeper into that, later.

What if you don't need carbohydrates at all?

Can you live without them?

**Can you live without them and still be healthy?**

# THE QUESTION I WOULD RATHER ASK,

# IF YOU CAN BE HEALTHIER WITHOUT THEM,

# WOULDN'T YOU WANT TO BE?

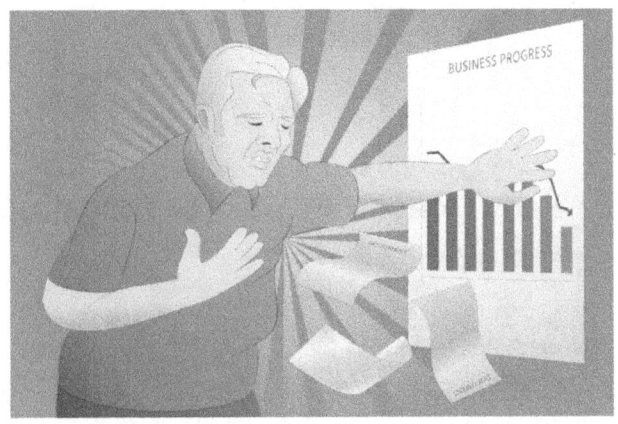

## ABSOLUTELY!

I can tell you right now, you can actually live healthier without them. I can tell you that you can live much easier without them. I can tell you that I live with much less pain without them and you too, can live with less pain without them. I can tell you that you'll have fewer headaches without them, I don't have headaches anymore. I can tell you that you won't have digestive problems anymore and I can tell you that most importantly, you can save your brain and actually make it work better, without them. Yes, I did say brain. I'll show you in article 4 how bread takes away any kind of dignity you've ever had because bread eats up your brain.

Does this mean that you misled in the past, when you were told that they had to be the largest portion of your diet? to eat them in excess? What was it Tony the Tiger always said, "they're Grrreeeaaat"?

What you're about to discover, is what the industry doesn't want you to know. They've taken steps to cover up this information and disprove it, by producing studies of their own trying to build up the benefit of these foods, they're selling.

I'm going to show you the science behind what their food is doing to you. Examine the evidence, analyze and assess the information, then you be the judge. I think, it's time for a cure, a time to put a stop to all the drugs, just to treat the symptoms, of what this food does to you.

## Your Body Does Not Need Carbohydrates.

You especially don't need them in the amounts that people everywhere are eating them. By everywhere, I mean everywhere. No place can be found where carbs are not a major part of the diet. To narrow down the problem with carbs, this article and entire book, deals entirely with the high starchy carbs you find in all cereal grains, primarily wheat, corn, barley, and rye because of the gluten that comes with it. But that's only part of it, which we'll talk about later in greater detail, because when you ingest gluten, you also take in gliadin. This is the part of wheat that can cause brain damage. That's something else that we'll talk about later, in greater detail when we look at how carbs have the capacity to shrink your brain. But this entails all grains including oats and rice, quinoa, and even legumes,  because of their ability to fluctuate blood glucose levels. All foods made from grains are dangerous foods to be eating on a regular basis and you as a consumer have a right to know exactly what this food is doing to your body. In this case, what you don't know, is stealing your brain and killing you slowly, painfully and expensively. You deserve better than what's being fed to you by the food industrial complex.

We should start with why you should limit your carbohydrate intake to as little as possible. For starters,  to save your brain and ensure yourself better health, lower weight and most importantly, less illness and disease throughout your life. Secondly, to reduce your your pain levels by reducing inflammation. Thirdly, to reduce headaches of any nature. and fourthly, to get better sleep. The full gamut of benefits is really much greater and is covered in the benefits articles, a *Life Without Carbs* and *My Life Without Carbs* in **part III breaking the addiction.**

Because your body can't burn carbohydrates (sugars), it has to turn them into fat, so they can used for fuel. Your body burns fat, not carbs. It actually likes fat so much, it would much rather have it spoon fed to it rather than make its own. The problem with using carbs to supply your fat, is that the fat it turns into, is not a good fat. Most of it gets stored instead of being used, and this is where the problem begins. It's the consumption of this starchy food that leads to the massive amounts of weight gain that everyone who eats it, experiences. But then, most of you already know this. It's just impossible to quit eating it, because of the **addictive** nature of the sticky, icky, gooey, gluey .sugar that's in all carbs.

**Time for a disclaimer;**

Not all people are subject to this weight gain from cereal grains, only about 90% of us are. That means, about 10% of the population have no intolerances to wheat, gluten or any of the components that come with it. That also means that for 90% of us, we do have an intolerance to it. That means, for 90% of us, we express an allergic reaction to it. The problem with that is, the allergic reaction we experience is weight gain and inflammation, and this damage happens, whether it's wanted or not. Anyone of us who has any kind of an intolerance to wheat, gluten or any other components of this grain will express this *'expansion'* and inflammation, when we eat it.

## Whether you want to accept it or not, carbs are dangerous.

I know you don't want to accept this, but bear with me, it's necessary for you to know what you're putting in your body and what it's doing to you. Even the smallest amount causes your body distress. This is why we shouldn't be eating this food to begin with, remember, (bread = carbs = sugar=glucose);

# For the short list,

## Carbs are responsible for;

1. Obesity

2. Type 2 diabetes

3. Celiac Disease

4. Epileptic seizures

5. Peripheral Neuropathy

6. Dementia and brain damage (type 3 diabetes)

7. Hypertension (High blood pressure)

8. Cardio Vascular and Heart disease

9. Most gastrointestinal disorders

10. A majority of cancers

11. Increase of LDL particles ("bad" cholesterol)

12. Arthritis (Primary contributor)

13. Emotional disorders by robbing you of control of your hormones

14. Sinus Headaches, Tension Headaches, Migraine Headaches

15. Tooth Decay

16. AGEs that age you quicker than any other influence (even more than stress)

The only way they can do this is because they're as addictive as heroin, cocaine, tobacco and alcohol. But they're also as just as deadly.

For the longer list, read **Wheat Belly** and **Grain Brain.** They'll fully explain what these carbs do to you as well as how they do it.

Let's take a closer look, though, at the these manifestations that not only can, but do occur from digesting this food.

- **Type 2 diabetes** is caused primarily by obesity and carbs play a major part in obesity. Carbs cause diabetes because of their need for insulin to be turned into fat so the body can use it. This is the beginning of a downhill spiral that forces the body to make adjustments that it would never have to do, if it were on a diet of protein and fats instead of carbohydrates. Because carbs have to be broken down to their most basic sugar, glucose to be used as a fuel, the glucose flows through your blood stream before it can be metabolized on a cellular level, to be used for that fuel. Glucose needs insulin, to be turned into fat to be digested, to use for energy. Glucose cannot enter the cell without insulin to turn it into fat. The problem is, most of the glucose, after it gets turned into fat, gets stored as fat in any one of the multitude of fat cells on your body. This takes place in the visceral fat (fat around the internal organs) first and foremost, where it's the most dangerous. The more carbs you eat, the more insulin your body needs to metabolize those carbs and with a body full of sugar, you need a lot of insulin to turn all those sugars into fat. After processing a diet full of high carbohydrate food over your lifetime, your body starts to have problems, manufacturing enough insulin, so you can continue to digest the carbs you continue to eat. Because your insulin production can't keep up with your carb intake, the sugar doesn't get turned into fat and stays in your blood stream as sugar. It begins to build up in your blood system, you become diabetic and this is the start of that downhill spiral. Hence the name insulin dependent diabetes or type two diabetes. If you were to remove the carbs, you'd remove the excess blood glucose. If you remove the glucose from the equation, you remove the diabetes. If you take away the carbs, you take away the obesity and excess glucose. Can it really be that simple? Duh! Thank you Dr Davis! I think it is a cure.
- **Peripheral Neuropathy** "Peripheral neuropathy (PN) is damage to, or disease, affecting the nerves, which may impair sensation, movement, gland or organ function, or other aspects of health, depending on the type of nerve affected." Wikipedia says, "It is important to recognize that glucose levels in the blood may spike to nerve-damaging levels after eating, even though fasting blood sugar levels and average blood glucose levels may still remain below normal levels (currently they typically are considered below 100 mg/dL for fasting blood plasma and 6.0%

for HGBA1c, the test commonly used to measure average blood glucose levels over an extended period). Studies have shown that many of the cases of peripheral small fiber neuropathy with typical symptoms of tingling, pain, and loss of sensation in the feet and hands are due to glucose intolerance before a diagnosis of diabetes or pre-diabetes. Such damage often is reversible, particularly in the early stages, with changes in diet, exercise, and weight loss." According to Dr Davis, "A common cause of peripheral neuropathy is diabetes. High blood sugars occurring repeatedly over several years damage the nerves in the legs, causing reduced sensation (thus allowing a diabetic to step on a thumbtack without knowing it), diminished control over blood pressure and heart rate, and sluggish emptying of the stomach (diabetic gastro paresis), among other manifestations of a nervous system gone haywire." He goes on to say, "Of 35 gluten-sensitive patients with peripheral neuropathy who were tested positive for the antigliadin antibody, the twenty-five participants on a wheat-and gluten-free diet improved over one year, while the ten control participants who did not remove wheat and gluten deteriorated." and " Formal studies of nerve conduction gluten-consuming group were also performed, demonstrating improved nerve conduction in the wheat-and gluten-free group, and deterioration in the wheat- and gluten-consuming group." Does anyone else see a smoking gun in these studies?

- **Celiac disease** "Celiac disease is caused by a reaction to gliadin, a prolamin (gluten protein) found in wheat, and similar proteins found in the crops of the tribe Triticeae (which includes other common grains such as barley and rye)." Gluten which is Latin for "glue" is a protein composite that acts as an adhesive material, holding flour together to make bread products, including crackers, baked goods, pasta and pizza dough. Made up primarily of gluten (amylose and amylopectin), it's this dough that likes to gum up things. Remember the last time you pigged out on pizza? Remember the indigestion? You think, that came from the sauce? Think again. Think amylose.

- **Dementia** and **Brain Damage** "Wheat is associated with dementia and brain dysfunction, triggering an immune response that infiltrates memory and mind." Dr. William Davis explains it best in his best seller, Wheat Belly, "In one particularly disturbing Mayo Clinic study of thirteen patients with the recent diagnosis of celiac disease, dementia was also diagnosed. Of those thirteen, frontal lobe biopsy (yes, brain biopsy) or postmortem examination of the brain failed to identify any other pathology beyond that associated with wheat gluten exposure. Prior to death or biopsy, the most common symptoms were memory loss, the inability to perform simple arithmetic, confusion, and change in personality. Of the thirteen, nine died due to progressive impairment of brain function." Yes: fatal dementia from wheat. Dr Perlmutter explains it in more detail in *Grain Brain.* If you want to join all the other seniors who are all losing their minds to Alzheimer's disease or dementia of any sort, all you have to do is to continue to eat your bread, pasta, crackers, pancakes, donuts, tortillas and other wheat products and you'll be right there with everyone else. When was the last time you misplaced your keys, couldn't remember somebody's name or forgot something? But look on the bright side of it, if you want to keep eating your donuts, you can, as long as you don't mind that you won't get to bathe yourself after a while, because you'll soon have it done for you. I talk more about why this happens in article 3, How carbs cause AGEs, your ticket to diabetes, Alzheimer's disease, cancer, heart disease and more.

- **Heart disease** (cardiovascular disease) has too many risk factors to list here, because there are many kinds of cardiovascular disease, but one of the biggest of concern, is the excess sugar in the blood (diabetes), as well obesity (excess weight the body needs to supply blood to), as well as the high blood pressure and the high amount of plaque in the blood due to the glycation of cholesterol thanks to the extra sugar in the blood. *"It is estimated that 90% of Heart disease is preventable."* All the causes listed here are caused by eating wheat. Life Insurance agents have to ask 4 times the standard premium to submit an application for a policy on anyone who has both diabetes and high blood pressure, because of the high underwriting risk. If they want a policy, they have to pay 4 times the standard premium because of their condition. And the condition is preventable. What's keeping you from declaring your independence? Addiction?

- **Multitudes of gastrointestinal disorders** are provoked by gumming up your digestive system with the gluten that comes with all wheat, especially the high gluten bread and pizza dough. Amylose, the sugar in wheat, is little more than glue. All this glue sticks to the walls of your intestines blocking the digestion of other foods as well as itself. Everyone I know who loves to consume their daily pastries, pastas, biscuits, rolls and crackers, already know about the cramps that build up in their stomachs, due to the amount of undigested food that can't get through the glue to get digested. This gluten, that's in wheat, barley, rye and almost every other variant of wheat, is the substance that causes all the damage to your digestive tract. This glue plays a major role in acid indigestion, acid reflux, heartburn, constipation, nausea, and even general stomach upset. With 10 different disorders of the digestive tract, gluten plays a gumming role in each one of them. You know the gas and bloating you get, sometimes after a meal? Guess what? Yeah, the major cause of that can be tracked to carbs. And it's not even included in the above list. I can't help but wonder why people continue to eat this pseudo food. I keep finding OTC medicine, that I've been purchasing over the years, just to combat, excess gas and bloating, acid indigestion, acid reflux, nausea, constipation, diarrhea, and worse yet ulcers. I don't use any of it anymore. All of these_manifestations could be curbed with the reduction of wheat and grains in your diets. I did it with mine. You can do it with yours. That gurgling you just heard from your stomach, was that your stomach telling you to get your act together, and curb the carb intake?

- **Cancer** gets its assist from the excess sugar that's continuously circulating in your blood. It keeps your ph levels in an acidic range which is an invitation to illness and disease. **Acidosis** is not something you want to have to deal with, with all the problems that it can produce. "Healthy human-arterial blood pH varies between 7.35 and 7.45. Changes in the pH of arterial blood (and therefore the extracellular fluid) outside this range result in irreversible cell damage." Cancer loves it when your blood ph levels go into acidosis from the amount of sugar, carbs dump into your blood. This is what leaves your body open for attack, from a multitude of illnesses and diseases, cancer only being one of them. Worse than the acidic *PH*, is the glycation of cholesterol and all the plaque it generates. A more complicated explanation of how carbs cause cancer is in the article about how *Carbs and Cancer Go Together Like Beetle and Juice*. Again, if cancer gets an assist from carbs, doesn't it make sense that if you took away the carbs, you'd, at the least, hamper the disease's, progression, if not stop it altogether. Can it be that simple? Can you give me a reason why you shouldn't try it and find out? If you have a reason, it's being demanded by your addiction.

- **Epileptic seizures** "A peculiar syndrome of temporal lobe seizures unresponsive to seizure medications and triggered by calcium deposition in a part of the temporal lobe called the hippocampus (responsible for forming new memories) has been associated with both celiac disease and gluten sensitivity (positive antigliadin antibodies and HLA markers without intestinal disease)." What Wikipedia is saying here is that you don't have to have Celiac disease to experience the brain damage that bread causes. All you have to have, is an intolerance of any sort, to gluten.

- **Arthritis** is a disease of inflammation, which is aggravated by wheat more than anything else, because of the amount of sugars it dumps into the blood stream. Few other sources of sugar are higher than bread and wheat products....not even table sugar. Arthritis is caused by inflammation. Inflammation is influenced by the amount of glucose in your blood, which in influenced by the amount of carbs you eat. Again, can it be that simple? Remove the carbs and you can ease, if not eliminate, it's influence on Arthritis.

- **Emotional Disruption and Disorder** takes place every time you ingest this food, in any form it's ingested, this is directly due to the to the changes your hormones go through because of the fluctuations in your blood glucose, caused by the consumption of wheat and grain foods. Blood sugars go up, moods rise. blood sugars go down, moods depress. It's that simple. The point I want to bring up, is it's the rise and fall of your blood sugars that have the biggest impact on your hormones and your emotional health. This in itself leads to behavior that, many times, should never occur in the first place. And it would never occur in the first place, if it weren't for the abundance of this food in our diet. Behavior like violence, bred by anger and antagonism, runs rampant where this food is commonplace in the diet. Both of these emotions are influenced as much, if not more than anything else, by the foods we eat. I submit that these fluctuations in emotional levels, are due to the changes in blood glucose, in all who

11

eat this food, and have been influenced by it. The hormonal changes this food puts your body through is under full control of what you eat. If you remove the wheat and grains, you control your hormones, yourself and remove the influence. If you remove the influence, you can easier retain your senses. It's that simple. Behavior driven by fear, is quite possibly the biggest danger our society faces, and this "staple" food source is a major cause in driving this behavior, because of is palatable nature. Sugar tastes good. People love to eat it. Mass consumption of it alters the emotional status of everyone who eats it, when their blood sugars fluctuate. It's these fluctuations that cause a large majority of the abhorrent behavior that pervades society everywhere. It's these fluctuations combined with the influence of mass media that are driving most of the terrorism in the world today. This theft of your emotional control, is what makes you a slave to corporate influence and subject to their desires, not your desires. How long going to allow them to retain control of your emotions?

- **Addiction** According to Dr Davis, "There is no doubt: For some people, wheat is addictive." It has to do with the effect it has on our neurotransmitters and neuropeptides , primarily Serotonin and Endorphins." Endorphins ("endogenous morphine") are endogenous opioid neuropeptides." They're the feel good neuropeptides . This is the same neuropeptide that's activated by alcohol, tobacco, heroin, cocaine, marijuana and all other substances of an addictive nature, that give you the '*morphine*' feeling. I submit this food is addictive to everyone who eats it except for the 10% of those who have no intolerances to it. When was the last time, you had to have something to eat? What was it, you hungered for? How long was it before you had eaten the previous time? How long can you go without eating? I often go 18 hours a day eating no more than 1 small piece of cheese, because of my keto diet. Can you?

- **Headaches** Headaches are primarily a manifestation of inflammation. Only one thing can create the inflammation that creates headaches and that's grains and sugar (glucose). I know this from experience. If carbs from grains really are responsible for headaches, doesn't that mean, if you take away the carbs, you'd take away the headaches? (it worked for me)

- **Tooth Decay** They rob You Of Your teeth. Ask any archaeologist, The appearance of rotten teeth marked the beginning of the agricultural age in our ancient history. It marked our move from being hunter-gatherers, to farmers. Even though this transition was one of the first moves into civilization, It also served to introduce our bodies to the ravages of carbohydrate nutrition. Fortunately, for our ancestors sake, it wasn't as dangerous then, as it is, now, as it hadn't been genetically modified. The wheat that was grown then was unmodified einkorn. It didn't rob us of our senses, then, because it didn't fluctuate blood sugars to the extent that all wheat and grain products, do today. But it still damaged the body. Any archeologist will tell you that. Whatever was eaten had more of the fiber left in it to slow down the absorption of sugars into the system. They didn't fluctuate the blood glucose, in the massive ways they do today. Even though they still caused the diseases, then, they weren't nearly as severe as they are, today. I submit, that it is this sudden fluctuation in sugars, that is causing 88% of all illnesses and diseases, that we have to deal with in our modern society. That, in itself, makes us victims of our own advancement, going back to the start of civilization. But, that's only looking at the past, at the reason why we're ingesting this food that ruins our teeth. Why it does that, most of you already know. It can be summed up in one word, sugar. Sugar rots teeth. Not meat, not cheese, not eggs, not fat, nothing that we consume rots teeth like carbohydrates do. The gluten that we love so much, makes it stick to our teeth, and this is where it begins to do its damage. The sugars work their way into the enamel of your teeth and the decay begins. You brush it away, you floss it away, and you do the best you very can, to keep your teeth as clean as possible. And when you make it to your 75 birthday, you pat yourself on the back, for still having all of your teeth. Or, do you? Have there been times when you couldn't brush and floss? Do you brush every time you take a sip of a sweet drink, or a drink of alcohol? All the sugar contained in those liquids, swirls around your mouth for hours and hours, working on decaying your teeth. Remove the sugar, remove the decay. It's that simple.
- **AGEs** Carbs are the root cause of aging due to the **A**dvanced **G**lycation **E**ndproducts, that they cause. This factor is at the root of so many disorders and diseases, that it deserves an article of its own.

Read *AGEs, your ticket to diabetes, heart disease, dementia, Alzheimer's Disease, Cancer and More,* coming up, to learn exactly what damage they are capable of.

**With all of these ailments, illnesses, diseases, disorders, afflictions, and discomfort being caused by carbs,**

**The questions I keep asking myself,**

**Who in their right mind would ever agree to submit themselves to this torture, by eating them?**

# THOSE WHO DON'T KNOW THAT THEY DO!

Most of us know that sugar is bad for us, but what too many don't want to fully recognize, is that carbs are sugar. With bread being the most popular carb we eat, every time we eat bread, we know that we're eating carbs, but we don't want to equate those carbs with sugar, while in all actuality they are. If Sugar Kills, Carbs Kill. In this case the bread is worse than sugar.

**WE KNOW THAT SUGAR KILLS, BUT WE DON'T WANT TO LISTEN TO THAT SONG BECAUSE OF OUR ADDICTION TO IT.**

All of the manifestations listed above have been documented in several publications, but they've seldom been presented for review and examination, to the medical community. Not until Dr's Davis' and Perlmutter's books, *Wheat Belly* and *Grain Brain,* came forth to warn us about the atrocities, this supposedly nutritious food has been doing to us, did I even know I was eating something that is so deviously dangerous (at least to the 90% of us, who have an intolerance and are allergic to it).

This, in my estimation, is the biggest problem. Most people **are** allergic to it. I estimate that more than 90% of the population have some sort of intolerance(s) to wheat, gluten or the gliadin that's in the wheat. That says, that more than 90% of the people are allergic to flour and everything that it comes in, bread, pasta, crackers, cereals like Wheaties, Wheat Germ, *or* Special K (to name just a few). That also means that any breaded chicken, shrimp, veal, all breaded fried appetizers, all pastries, all nutrition bars, all cereal bars, anything that has any percentage of wheat or wheat substance in it, are off limits too. The list is too long, even for the length of this article. The question this begs, is why is this food still advertised as being healthy?

If 90% of the population, (as I speculate) are allergic to wheat, then 90% of the population is addicted to it. It's what makes us allergic to it, that makes it addictive to us and that's where the danger lies. Article 14 explains why. This also explains why I made the claim, at the beginning of this article, you do not need carbohydrates.

If you're one of the 90% who are allergic to them, you'd be much better off without them. With as many problems as this food brings with it, it makes absolutely no sense to continue eating it except to feed your addiction. So this brings us to our next problem, breaking our addiction to them.

The question this conjures then, how do we stop eating them? How do we get this food that's been such an important part of our diet since time immemorial, out of our diet? For that, you'll have to continue on to Article 13, *How to cut back.*

If anybody feels that any of these conclusions are nothing more than opinion, my challenge to you is, prove me wrong, that's your addiction speaking and I invite you to research any and all statements, facts, data of any sort, or links, that I've provided in these articles, to invalidate anything. I'll even go to the extent to challenge anyone to prove me wrong, in any of my statements. It will generate a good civil discussion, and that's something I can look forward to, anytime.

My sincere wish, is that everyone who reads these pages verifies and validates what they read. Only then will they know that the information contained within this site is 100% valid. Maybe then, all who read this, will change their behavior and in turn, change the behavior of the whole world.

My challenge to you, is to give a low carb diet a try, for 2 months. If you don't see any benefit after just 2 months, of abstinence, go back to your high carb diet. But please, prepare yourself to suffer the consequences. The attempt must be an honest attempt, with absolutely no cheating (no carbs), for this to work. Any deviation, will not let your body go into ketosis and that's what's important.

# YOU HAVE TO LOOK AT IT

# LIKE YOUR LIFE DEPENDS ON IT,

# BECAUSE, IT DOES. NOTHING ELSE IS AS

# IMPORTANT AS YOUR HEALTH AND

# NOTHING INFLUENCES THAT MORE

# THAN WHAT YOU CONSUME

# Article 2

## Sugar; America's Deadliest Addiction

### Confessions From a Reformed Carboholic

Sugar, I love it. I grew up loving it. Because I grew up loving it, I'm now addicted to it. It's an addiction that was forced upon me by our food industrial complex, telling my mother that she had to feed it to me. She fed me this food to keep me healthy. That was 60 years ago. I'm paying the price for that now, with my arthritis. I was paying the price for it just 30 months ago, by carrying 60 lbs more than what I carry right now, and being borderline diabetic.

My sisters are paying the price for it now. They both are obese and diabetic. My father has always exercised. He's always been able to burn off the excess glucose, until he was about 35. Since then, he's always jogged every day, ever since I was in 7th grade, but even he couldn't run away from this.

My mother, in trying to be the best mother and wife she could be, went along with what the FDA and the ADA told her because she wanted to do what was right for her family. She wanted to do what she was told to by our government. Guidelines from the ADA telling her that grains needed to be at the base of her all of her meals was what drove her to do this to our family. This is what doomed us to our current list of ailments, ailments like obesity and diabetes, arthritis, cancer, stomach ailments galore, and now, side effects from treatment for those ailments. It all comes along with a carbohydrate diet because all carbs break down into glucose.

Because sugar addiction is America's biggest addiction, that makes it, its worst addiction. It's an addiction that everybody grew up with and into. It's an addiction that's been with us for as long as we've been eating it. It's an addiction that's become far worse than it's ever been, since we've been eating it over its 10,000 year history. It's an addiction that's built scores of empires, and then tore them all down.

This addiction is far worse than any other addiction that plagues America. Whether it be today, yesterday or tomorrow, this addiction is the worst that Man has ever faced or may ever face. This is simply due to its propensity to expand its influence across the whole world. It's also driven by the greed of those condemned to this addiction. Their desire to feed their own addiction drives them to impose this addiction on the rest of the world, simply so they can make an extra buck.

This addiction is at the root of almost every known form of dementia, heart disease, diabetes, as well as everything that comes along with that, like cancers, cardiovascular diseases. The list is endless because glucose's worst instigator of inflammation, AGEs, or glycation is at the base of an arm long list of disorders.

All of these disorders can be curbed simply by curbing carbohydrate consumption but addiction keeps this from happening. That's why fighting this addiction in particular is so important. It's life saving at its simplest, just remove contaminating factors from the food source and the diseases cannot manifest themselves.

The contaminating factor in this case? You guessed it, sugar. Sugar addiction is leading our society to the brink of destruction because of the nature of its addiction and what it does to the body. Its continued use only leads to discomfort and death. It's only redeeming factor is that it tastes good and satiates quickly. This is what makes it so deadly, though.

That's sad. I know it, I have to live with it too. I can't have what I love, what I've been addicted to. I have to say no, to stay healthy. So do you. I know that's exactly the opposite of what you've been told, but what you were told is wrong. For us it's dead wrong. It should have never been pushed upon us, to eat it in the quantities that it's been promoted.

But pushed upon us it was and is. We bought it then and we're still buying it now. We bought into it big time and we're paying for it now.

This is evidenced by the proliferation of Alzheimer's disease. How many lives does it have to take, before people wake up? How many families does it have to destroy, before people realize what few doctors are trying to tell us? Unfortunately, only a few, Dr Davis and Dr Perlmutter.

We need clinics for sugar addiction and they should be financed by the food industrial complex that imposed this diet on the people who now suffer from the consequences of it. The administration of the clinic though, should be done by trained medical professionals, because this is an addiction and should be treated as such.

Is this something that should be investigated? Should an industry be held accountable for the ruse that's been pulled on the American people, and now the world? The ruse that this is healthy food, when it's really not? Why are they still allowed to claim that it's healthy? Why are they still, allowed to advertise that it's healthy? It's clearly not, and it's clearly at the root of almost all of the deadliest diseases, that we're actively fighting right now. Diseases like Atherosclerosis, Endocarditis and Hypertensive heart disease. That's just the CVD's. We haven't even covered the cancers, or dementias. Those lists are much longer.

Can anyone tell me why this is still allowed to be advertised like it is today? It starts with what's put in baby food for starches and fillers and sweeteners. These fillers satiate babies quickly often putting them right to sleep after a short burst of energy. This is the first indication of sugar addiction and it starts at a young age. This is done for a purpose. That purpose is to addict you to its lure, so you'll buy into it when you're an adult.

It continues with your introduction to breakfast cereals and the load of sugars they carry when you see them advertised with the Saturday morning cartoons. I can remember for commercials for Sugar Pops, Sugar Frosted Flakes, and Captain Crunch. It starts young, real young and continues through your youth with candy and soda, and into your adult years with bread and baked goods (cakes, crackers, cookies).

It's been forced upon us. Nobody has had a choice in this addiction and that is what makes it so lethal. That also makes it profitable for the Pharmaceutical industry. This is what scares me. The Pharmaceutical industry used to be owned by the same industry the provided the crop seed for the farmers that grew the grain that provided the flour to bake all of those loaves of bread that causing so much disease.

It's almost the perfect scam. Sell crop seed to farmers that's been genetically modified, so that it feeds your customer base, food that will require them, in the future to purchase medications from your other companies. How convenient we've made it for this industry to take our money. We should be ashamed.

We would be ashamed if we knew that this was done intentionally, especially if it was done for nothing more than profit. That is why this is something that should be investigated. Regardless of how long it takes, we need to know who is responsible. This is a lesson that cannot be lost. Like every other study done on these concerns, we cannot allow this to be swept under the rug. The only way we can prevent this in the future we is if we hold these companies accountable, now.

We cannot allow our society to continue to celebrate our addiction to glucose as we do now and have in the past. We've always enjoyed celebrating our addiction, because we never treated it as an addiction and thus never looked at it in that way. Yet, it is an addiction, and it's a bad addiction, as displayed throughout these pages. It's consumption is more detrimental to our health than any other source of damage, whether it be stress, smoking, sun damage or environmental pollution. If we didn't have the carb addiction, every other source of damage could and would be much easier tolerated.

For 1,000s of years, we've been treating the symptoms of the diseases and disorders of this addiction. Because of our addiction, we've never looked at the prospect of eliminating the true cause completely. When a whole society is addicted to a staple that they've eaten their whole lives, how does one tell the truth about something that is so important to everyone on the planet? How does one tell everyone that what they're eating is killing them slowly, expensively, painfully, and worst of all, without any dignity, because of all the lost memories from brain damage? How does one tell a whole society that a staple that they've lived on for close to 10,000 years has been, and continues to be, the one food that creates more disease and illness than any other one food in their diet? How does a world break their addiction, when the addicted are the majority of the world and only 5% of that population can recognize their addiction?

Dr Perlmutter is trying to tell the people and continues to do so. I honestly feel that he thinks as I do, that if we don't dispel the consumption of these foods, our society is doomed. From what I've learned, since I've broken the addiction, I see a collapse, due to out of control emotions, due to the wild glucose swings in the blood, making people under the control of a carbohydrate diet, under the control of those who impose this diet on the American public. It's in their interest to keep America addicted and the best way they can do this, is to tell you that it's healthy and that it's what you need to keep your body healthy.

Only those who want to buy their pharmaceuticals, from them in the future, are the ones who should be buying their food products now, because eventually, they will.

By following what little advice I offer, to curb your carbs dramatically and as completely as possible, you can dramatically slow down if not eliminate many of the disorders and diseases within these pages. If it can't eliminate your disease, it will reduce the expression of your disorder. If it doesn't cure you, it will definitely extend your life. My goal is to extend it a minimum of 20 years. I would like to see everyone live to be 100 years old, or more. I know this diet lifestyle can do that (depending on your age and degree of addiction of course). To Know this yourself, though? You have to try it. You'll only know, for sure, after you try it

# Part II

## **The Evidence**

# Article 3
## HOW CARBS ARE RESPONSIBLE FOR AGEs, YOUR TICKET TO DIABETES, ALZHEIMER'S DISEASE, CANCER, HEART DISEASE AND MORE

AGEs are the, most influential, factor in what makes us old and are responsible for the majority of the illness and disease that we live with today. Dr Perlmutter explains it much better in his book *Grain Brain* in chapter 4, about Advanced Glycation End-products;

"Glycation is the biochemical term for the bonding of sugar molecules to proteins, fats, and amino acids; the spontaneous reaction that causes the sugar molecule to attach itself is sometimes referred to as the Maillard reaction. Louis Camille Maillard first described this process in the early 1900s. Although he predicted that this reaction could have an important impact on medicine, not until 1980 did medical scientists turn to it when trying to understand diabetic complications and aging."

"This process forms advanced glycation end products (commonly shortened, appropriately, to AGEs), which cause protein fibers to become misshapen and inflexible. To get a glimpse of AGEs in action, simply look at someone who is prematurely aging—someone with a lot of wrinkles, sagginess, discolored skin, and a loss of radiance for their age. What you're seeing is the physical effect of proteins hooking up with renegade sugars, which explains why AGEs are now considered key players in skin aging. Or check out a chain-smoker: The yellowing of the skin is another hallmark of glycation. Smokers have fewer antioxidants in their skin, and the smoking itself increases oxidation in their bodies and skin. So they cannot combat the by-products of normal processes like glycation because their bodies' antioxidant potential is severely weakened and, frankly, overpowered by the volume of oxidation. For most of us, the external signs of glycation show up in our thirties, when we've accumulated enough hormonal changes and environmental oxidative stress, including sun damage." "Glycation is an inevitable fact of life, just like inflammation and free radical production to some degree. It's a product of our normal metabolism and fundamental in the aging process. We can even measure glycation using technology that illuminates the bonds formed between sugars and proteins. In fact, dermatologists are well versed in this process. With Visia complexion-analysis cameras, they can capture the difference between youth and age just by taking a fluorescent image of children and comparing it to the faces of older adults. The children's faces will come out very dark, indicating a lack of AGEs, whereas the adults' will beam brightly as all those glycation bonds light up."

This is inflammation at its core. It's these particles that are responsible for inflammation. These free radicals roaming around your body wreaking havoc wherever they go, arthritis in your joints, or stiffening and clogging your arteries with the plaque that they're  the foundation of. This is the same plaque the that builds up in your heart and brain and other organs.

According to Wikipedia; "In human nutrition and biology, advanced glycation end products, known as AGEs, are substances that can be a factor in the development or worsening of many degenerative diseases, such as diabetes, atherosclerosis, chronic renal failure, and Alzheimer's disease."

Wikipedia goes on to say, "These harmful compounds can affect nearly every type of cell and molecule in the body and are thought to be one factor in aging and in some age-related chronic diseases. They are also believed to play a causative role in the blood-vessel complications of diabetes mellitus. AGEs are seen as speeding up oxidative damage to cells and in altering their normal behavior."

The questions this conjures, is, whatever could cause these damaging substances? They're a normal part of aging, but what amplifies their behavior, is a part of our diet that's been with us forever, grain based carbohydrates plain and simple. I understand why this is hard for some of you to accept, so we'll go through all of the effects they cause and look at what role, wheat and gluten play in each part.

### AGEs have a range of pathological effects, such as:

- Increased vascular permeability.
- Increased arterial stiffness - (leads to hypertension)

- Inhibition of vascular dilation by interfering with nitric oxide.
- Oxidizing LDL. - (increasing plaque production)
- Binding cells—including macrophage, endothelial, and mesangial—to induce the secretion of a variety of cytokines. (The foundation of inflammation.)
- Enhanced oxidative stress. - (foundation of CVDs and cancer)

Oxidative stress is caused by "Glycation (sometimes called non-enzymatic glycosylation) is the result of typically covalent bonding of a protein or lipid molecule with a sugar molecule, such as fructose or glucose, without the controlling action of an enzyme."

"Some AGEs are benign, but others are more reactive than the sugars they are derived from, and are implicated in many age-related chronic diseases such as cardiovascular diseases (the endothelium, fibrinogen, and collagen are damaged), Alzheimer's disease (amyloid proteins are side-products of the reactions progressing to AGEs), cancer (acrylamide and other side-products are released), peripheral neuropathy (the myelin is attacked), and other sensory losses such as deafness (due to demyelination). This range of diseases is the result of the very basic level at which glycations interfere with molecular and cellular functioning throughout the body and the release of highly oxidizing side-products such as hydrogen peroxide."

Of all the factors responsible for AGEs, and their effects listed above, the two we're going to look at are oxidative stress and cytokines. The primary reason I want to examine these factors is because these two are responsible for what makes many carboholics look 70, when they're actually only 50. So, let's break down each part; we'll start with cytokines. If you haven't checked out what Wikipedia has to say about these destroyers of life, we'll do so now, right now.

"Cytokines are a broad and loose category of small proteins that are important in cell signaling. They are released by cells and affect the behavior of other cells. Cytokines are produced by a broad range of cells, including immune cells like macrophages, B lymphocytes, T lymphocytes and mast cells, as well as endothelial cells, fibroblasts, and various stromal cells; a given cytokine may be produced by more than one type of cell."

Cytokines like hormones, are cell signaling proteins that instruct other cells how to perform. Leptin signals the production of more leptin, to encourage the production of more fat, cytokines appear to be at the core of free radical damage, which can multiply at a much faster rate, because of the nature of free radicals. I believe that many cytokines are glycated proteins, which means they can end up being any kind of macrophage,   B lymphocytes, T lymphocytes or mast cell.

It really is a vicious cycle. This is where you need your anti-oxidants, which are produced through exercise and calorie restriction, which we talk about later. (These are truly life saving habits. More than life saving, they're life extending.)

Concerning cytokines though, "They act through receptors, and are especially important in the immune system; cytokines modulate the balance  between humoral and cell-based immune  responses,  and they regulate the maturation, growth, and responsiveness of particular cell populations. Some cytokines enhance or inhibit the action of other cytokines in complex ways. They are different from hormones, which are also important cell signaling molecules, in that hormones circulate in much lower concentrations and hormones tend to be made by specific kinds of cells." Of the different cell signaling proteins, hormones and cytokines, cytokines are the Mr Hyde to the Dr Jekyll of hormones. For whatever good hormones can do for you, most cytokines do that much damage when they're released into your body. These free radicals can be deadly. In larger concentrations, they are deadly.

"They are important in health and disease, specifically in host responses  to  infection,  immune  responses, inflammation, trauma, sepsis, cancer, and reproduction. A key focus of interest has been that cytokines in one of these two sub-sets tend to inhibit the effects of those in the other. Dysregulation of this tendency is under intensive  study  for  its  possible  role  in  the  pathogenesis  of autoimmune disorders. Several inflammatory cytokines are induced by oxidative stress. The fact that cytokines themselves trigger the release of other cytokines and also lead to increased oxidative stress makes them important in chronic inflammation, as well as other immune responses, such as fever and acute phase proteins of the liver."

If all this is the responsibility of cytokines, and cytokines cause oxidative stress, what role does the oxidative stress play in this equation? We know it leads to inflammation at the very least, but what else does it do?

"Oxidative stress reflects an imbalance between the systemic manifestation of reactive oxygen species and a biological system's ability to readily detoxify the reactive intermediates or to repair the resulting damage." Basically, this is the inability of the body, to be able to heal itself from the daily stresses of life.

If detoxify here, implies to ridding toxins from the body, it makes sense that the system's ability to detoxify will be compromised, when the toxin that's most abundant in the body is the residue of glucose combustion, done a cellular level. Glucose combustion residue is the spent fuel from lipids that come from fat made from glucose. That makes this residue as sticky as the lipid that created it, a lipid that was sticky. This is what I call dirty fat, because of its nature of being sticky. These are the lipids that cluster around Apolipoprotein B to form LDL particles. These particles are the true "bad cholesterol" and they're the worst kind of LDL particles to be feeding your cells. More about that in article 11.

"In humans, oxidative stress is thought to be involved in the development of Asperger syndrome, ADHD, cancer, Parkinson's disease, Lafora disease, Alzheimer's disease, atherosclerosis, heart failure, myocardial infarction, fragile X syndrome, Sickle Cell Disease, lichen planus, vitiligo, autism,[ infection, and chronic fatigue syndrome. However, reactive oxygen species can be beneficial, as they are used by the immune system as a way to attack and kill pathogens. Short-term oxidative stress may also be important in prevention of aging by induction of a process named mitohormesis."

We know now that oxidative stress is so bad for you in the long term, it's deadly, and yet good for you in the short term. So, what about the short term benefits? How do you achieve those? What do the short term benefits entail?

The short term benefits of oxidative stress, mitohormesis, comes mostly from exercise, but also from certain spices, like "curcumin from turmeric, green tea extract, silymarin (milk thistle), bacopa extract, DHA, sulforaphane (contained in broccoli), and ashwagandha".

"Short-term oxidative stress may also be important in prevention of aging by induction of a process named mitohormesis. "Short term oxidative stress also helps build up Nrf2 in your brain which can supercharge your production of antioxidants. According to Wikipedia, "Activation of Nrf2 results in the induction of many cytoprotective proteins."

Exercise is the best way to induce mitohormesis. But it can be found in curcumin also (as mentioned above) which can be found in turmeric, an important spice used extensively on the Indian subcontinent. This one little compound is so important in the proliferation of your antioxidants, that some drug companies, are trying to copy it with their own chemical versions, like, Tecfidera, Oltipraz, and Bardoxolone methyl, to name a few. It's that important. You can get it free, right now, by just exercising. Why wait for another drug?

Calorie restriction is another way to build up your anti-oxidants. This will build up more anti-oxidants in you than what you could ever eat or drink. We'll talk more about that later.

"One of the areas where the concept of hormesis has been explored extensively with respect to its applicability is aging. Since the basic survival capacity of any biological system depends on its homeostatic ability should result in the adaptive or hormetic response with various biological benefits. This idea has now gathered a large body of supportive evidence showing that repetitive mile stress exposure has anti-aging effects. Exercise is a paradigm for hormesis in this respect. Some of the mild stresses used for such studies on the application of hormesis in aging research and interventions are heat shock, irradiation, prooxidants, hypergravity and food restriction. Some other natural and synthetic molecules, such as medicinal herbs and curcumin from the spice turmeric have also been found to have hormetic beneficial effects. Such compounds which bring about their healthy beneficial effects by stimulating or by modulating stress response pathways in cells have been termed "hormetins". Hormetic interventions have also been proposed at the clinical level, with a variety of stimuli, challenges and stressful actions, that aim to increase the dynamical complexity of the biological systems in humans."

"Epidemiological data suggest that individuals with a low calorie intake may have a reduced risk of stroke and neurodegenerative disorders. There is a strong correlation between per capita food consumption and risk for Alzheimer's disease and stroke. Data from population-based case control studies showed that individuals with the lowest daily calorie intakes had the lowest risk of Alzheimer's disease and Parkinson's disease." Because "calorie restriction has been demonstrated in a variety of laboratory models to induce Nrf2 activation", it's as important as the exercise. "Nrf2 is a basic leucine zipper (bZIP) protein that regulates the expression of antioxidant proteins that protect against oxidative damage triggered by injury and inflammation."

When calories are reduced in the diets of lab animals, "they not only live longer, but also become remarkably resistant to the development of several cancers." This is according to Dr Perlmutter, in Grain Brain. Calorie restriction is close to impossible when you are a carboholic, on a carbohydrate diet. Every two hours or so you need another infusion of glucose into your system, to keep you going. Your hunger cycles force you into this repetitive behavior. You really have little choice in controlling it because of the drop in your sugar levels and the ensuing reaction of your hormones. A carboholic cannot stand the rigors and stress of fasting as easy as someone who's been on a keto diet for of any length of time. This is one of the biggest reasons that I remain on my MCT keto diet. If you're on a carbohydrate diet, your primary motivating factor is hunger. Mine is knowledge and a desire for more brainpower.

Roy Knight Jr

What's the best way to build up Nrf2 and protect your brain from the plaque of glycation? A diet high in fats, omega 3 fats in particular, MCT's are the best. MCTs like coconut oil, and a diet low in carbohydrates. Why? To me, it's simple, fats won't glycate other fats. Glycation occurs when glucose mixes with lipoproteins (cholesterol). It's sugars that glycate cholesterol. If, it's the glycation of cholesterol that leads to most illness and diseases, and building up Nrf2 in your brain can help protect you from that glycation, why wouldn't you want to build it up?

Dr. Perlmutter, says it better, in *Grain Brain* in chapter 5, where he explains the effect of antioxidant protection, and how we can generate more antioxidants, with our diet, than what we can ever ingest through drinking antioxidant beverages. He says, *"Several natural compounds that turn on antioxidant and detoxification pathways through activation of the Nrf2 system have been identified"*, which we talked about above.

To summarize; Carbs create AGEs; The "Glycation" end-products of AGEs are responsible for oxidative stress, dumping cytokines throughout your entire system to affect pretty much everything your blood flows through, including the arteries themselves.

"Oxidative stress is suspected to be important in neurodegenerative diseases including Lou Gehrig's disease (aka MND or ALS), Parkinson's disease, Alzheimer's disease, Huntington's disease, and Multiple sclerosis. Indirect evidence via monitoring biomarkers such as reactive oxygen species, and reactive nitrogen species production, antioxidant defense indicates oxidative damage may be involved in the pathogenesis of these diseases, while cumulative oxidative stress with disrupted mitochondrial respiration and mitochondrial damage are related with Alzheimer's disease , Parkinson's disease, and other neurodegenerative diseases. Oxidative stress is thought to be linked to certain cardiovascular disease, since oxidation of LDL in the vascular endothelium is a precursor to plaque formation. Oxidative stress also plays a role in the ischemic cascade due to oxygen reperfusion injury following hypoxia. This cascade includes both strokes and heart attacks. Oxidative stress has also been implicated in chronic fatigue syndrome. Oxidative stress also contributes to tissue injury following irradiation and hyperoxia as well as in diabetes, is likely to be involved in age-related development of cancer. The reactive species produced in oxidative stress can cause direct damage to the DNA and are therefore mutagenic, and it may also suppress apoptosis and promote proliferation, invasiveness and metastasis. Infection by Helicobacter pylori which increases the production of reactive oxygen and nitrogen species in human stomach is also thought to be important in the development of gastric cancer."

"Oxidative stress frees up cytokines to disrupt your biological balance, causing multiple diseases, like; Asperger syndrome, ADHD, cancer, Parkinson's disease, Lafora disease, Alzheimer's disease, atherosclerosis, heart failure, myocardial infarction, fragile X syndrome, Sickle Cell Disease, lichen planus, vitiligo, autism, infection, and chronic fatigue syndrome. "

AGEs can make you appear as much as 20 years older than what you actually are, because of this oxidative stress

They grey your hair. They wrinkle your skin. They take away your dignity by taking away your brain along with any ability it ever had, slowly, deliberately and very silently until it's too late (You literally won't know what hit you.)

## ECC (EXCESSIVE CARB CONSUMPTION), RESPONSIBLE FOR AGES, AGE YOU SEVERELY AND IS DEADLY

With all of these deadly consequences AGEs offer, why do people still continue to eat carbs and continue to suffer the effects of dealing with the long term effects of these things?

Short term effects are really beneficial, like increasing your auto immune system by ramping up your antioxidant production, protecting from all of the above diseases. If abstaining from carbs can bring you some of the short term effects, again, I have to ask myself, why do people still continue to eat carbs and continue to suffer the long term effects of these things? But then, I know the answer, Addiction!

# Article 4

## Curbing Carbs For Diabetes Control

**Diabetes is the Worst manifestation of carbohydrate addiction.**

**As carbs are the major influence in type 2 diabetes,**

**this article deals entirely with type 2 diabetes.**

Type 1 diabetes is an auto-immune disorder in which the pancreas is instructed not to produce insulin to convert glucose into fat, so it can be utilized, leaving excessive amounts of glucose to run rampant in the body. Although it has been speculated that glucose might play a part in type 1 diabetes by triggering certain hormones that trigger auto-immune responses, we're only going to deal with type 2 diabetes is this article.

Only because of the extra glucose in the blood stream, is this disorder called diabetes. In all actuality, type 2 diabetes is the result of carbohydrate overload, and should be called carbolism. I call it carbolism, simply because of its addictive nature, and how it acts upon the body in the same way that alcohol does. Alcohol is, after all, the same as a carbohydrate (sugar).

As described in *Carbs, The Newly Found Death Sentence;*

Type 2 diabetes is caused primarily by carrying extra fat on the body and carbs play a major part in that. Carbs cause type2 diabetes because of their need for insulin to be turned into fat so the body can use it. This is the beginning of a downhill spiral that forces the body to make adjustments that it would never have to do, if it were on a diet of protein and fats instead of carbohydrates. Because carbs have to be broken down to their most basic sugar, glucose to be used as a fuel, that glucose flows through your blood stream before it can be metabolized on a cellular level, to be used for that fuel. Glucose needs insulin, to be turned into fat to be digested, to use for energy. Glucose cannot enter the cell without insulin to turn it into fat. The problem is, most of the glucose, after it gets turned into fat, it gets stored as fat in any one of the multitude of fat cells on your body. This takes place in the visceral fat (fat around the internal organs) first and foremost, where it's the most dangerous. The more carbs you eat, the more insulin your body needs to metabolize those carbs and with a body full of sugar (carbs), you need a lot of insulin to turn all that glucose into fat. After processing a diet full of high carbohydrate food over your lifetime, your body starts to have problems, manufacturing enough insulin, so you can continue to digest the carbs you continue to eat. Because your insulin production can't keep up with your carb intake, the sugar doesn't get turned into fat and stays in your blood stream as sugar. It begins to build up in your blood system and you become diabetic. Hence the name insulin dependent diabetes or type two diabetes. Remove the carbs, remove the excess blood glucose. If you remove the glucose from the equation, you remove the diabetes. If you take away the carbs, you take away the obesity and excess glucose. Can it really be that simple?      Thank you, Dr Davis.

"Insulin induces HMG-CoA reductase activity, whereas glucagon diminishes HMC-CoA reductase activity. As glucagon production is stimulated by dietary protein ingestion, insulin production is stimulated by dietary carbohydrate ingestion. The rise of insulin is, in general, determined by the digestion of carbs into glucose and subsequent increase in serum glucose levels. In non-diabetics, glucagon levels are very low when insulin levels are high; however, those who have become diabetic no longer suppress glucagon output after eating."

This is why this disorder is called type 2 diabetes and it has little to do with type 1 diabetes except that it allows glucose to continue to flow in your blood without being turned into fat, allowing glycation to occur in a massive way. Type 1 diabetes is an auto-immune disease that shuts down the manufacture of insulin, by the pancreas, by destroying the cells where insulin is produced.

The fact that carbs are the only cause of type 2 diabetes, should be a warning to all who continue to eat this food. But what should alarm everyone, is what the excess glucose does, that carbs put into your system, because it's this excess glucose, that's so deadly. But then, we saw that in the discussion about AGEs.

**Glucose and cholesterol are the basic building blocks of plaque buildup in your system and it's this plaque, that kills.**

Cholesterol is formed by lipids (fat) clinging around protein cells called apolipoproteins. They come basically in two forms that make up high density and low density particles, the foundation of cholesterol in your blood. You can read about that in article 10 about *The Foundation of LDL Cholesterol; apolipoprotein B.*

It's excess fat in our bodies that form excess cholesterol in our bodies by providing the triglycerides to be formed into cholesterol. It's this excess cholesterol in the form of LDL particles that drives the fuel necessary to manifest any one of a multitude of illnesses, disorders, and diseases.

**When you combine these two destructive forces of glucose and fat or protein in the body, without an enzyme or signaling cell to tell it what to do, it's like two weather systems colliding. Havoc ensues.**

Plaque is by far the worst manifestation of diabetes and a carbohydrate diet. It happens when glucose molecules bind with fat, cholesterol or protein molecules, before they can be metabolized by your cells, and displays the true destructive force that glucose is responsible for, in and on your body.

According to Wikipedia, "there are seven different kinds of plaque, Amyloid, Atheroma, Dental plaque, Mucoid plaque, Pleural plaque, Senile plaques, Viral plaque." We're going to look at only 4 of these though.

By far the worst of the plaques caused by digesting wheat and gluten is amyloid plaque, because of all the diseases it has a role in. According to the NIH's, PMC;

1. "Amyloid fibril formation is considered to be a signature of neurodegenerative processes. The exact processes leading to cellular degeneration remain unknown although several amyloid-

involving mechanisms have been proposed. Amyloids occupy the extracellular space and destroy the structure of cells and tissues, amyloid fibrils destabilize cell membranes, Some proteins forming amyloids, for instance α-synuclein which contributes to the formation of intracellular Lewy bodies in Parkinson's disease, other proteins with an unordered structure are the IAPP in type II diabetes and β-amyloid in Alzheimer's disease. Such an unfolded structure allows the protein to be rather easily self-assembled into fibrils."

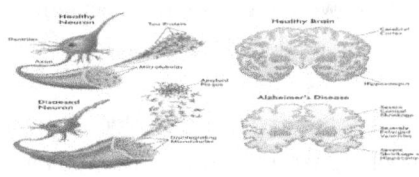

2.  "Atheromatous Plaques are basically plaques from fats and is the type of plaque that clogs up your artery walls. This is the type of plaque that causes atherosclerosis and leads to heart and cardio vascular disease."

3.  Dental plaque is caused by the excessive amount of sugar on the teeth, creating bacteria, causing decay.

4   "Senile plaques (also known as neuritic plaques, senile druse and brain druse) are extracellular deposits of amyloid beta in the grey matter of the brain. "

They cause Alzheimer's disease and dementia, and play a role in most every other cognitive disorder due to the way this plaque gums of the neurons in your brain.

This is why Type 3 diabetes is considered dementia or brain damage and this is the major reason you don't want to play around with type 2 diabetes, the next step is loss of your memories, and you won't even know it, as you won't realize it as it happens.

**Glucose and fat are responsible for plaque buildup**

Roy Knight Jr

You need both glucose and lipids flowing through your body to create plaque. The glucose attaches itself to a lipid (fat) molecule that has yet to be metabolized for energy, and glycates that lipid molecule. The lipids in this case are LDL cholesterol. Low density lipoproteins particles.

Because they float around in such loose form, they're easily attacked by any free flowing glucose in the system. This is the doom of maintaining a high amount of glucose in the body.

This is the beginning of plaque. Multiply this by the amount of carbohydrates your ingest every day. The result is exponentially worse than you would ever want to believe. The kind of plaque the carbs are turned into is dictated by the type of carb that made the lipid in the first place.

Plaque is by far the worst manifestation of a carbohydrate diet. It happens when glucose combines with any lipid, or protein cell without a signaling cell to tell it what to do and glycates that lipid or protein and it's here that it displays the true destructive force of glucose on your body. According to Wikipedia, there are seven different kinds of plaque, Amyloid, Atheroma, Dental plaque, Mucoid plaque, Pleural plaque, Senile plaques, Viral plaque. This displays the ultimate problem with getting protein and fats from a carbohydrate diet.

We're going to look deeper into only 5 of these. Pleural plaque deals with Mesothemiola, the cancer caused by exposure to asbestos. Nor are we going to examine viral plaques, as they're usually associated with viruses.

By far the worst of the plaques caused by digesting wheat and gluten is amyloid plaque, because of all the diseases it has a role in. According to the NIH's, PMC;

1.  1"Amyloid fibril formation is considered to be a signature of neurodegenerative processes. The exact processes leading to cellular degeneration remain unknown although several amyloid-involving mechanisms have been proposed. Amyloids occupy the extracellular space and destroy the structure of cells and tissues, amyloid fibrils destabilize

36

cell membranes, Some proteins forming amyloids, for instance α-synuclein which contributes to the formation of intracellular Lewy bodies in Parkinson's disease, other proteins with an unordered structure are the IAPP in type II diabetes and β-amyloid in Alzheimer's disease . Such an unfolded structure allows the protein to be rather easily self-assembled into fibrils."

2.  2 Atheromatous Plaques are basically macrophage cells containing lipids and cholesterol, and is the type of plaque that clogs up your artery walls. This is the type of plaque that causes atherosclerosis and leads to heart and cardio vascular disease. It is the root cause of high blood pressure.

3.  *"Mucoid plaque, a supposed thick coating of abnormal mucous material in the colon"* I don't have to wonder what create mucous in the colon. I know through experience, what creates mucous in the body. It's the sticky, gooey, gluey, yummy but deadly effects of a carbohydrate diet. The more carbs you eat, the worse your affliction and the sooner your demise.

4.  "Senile plaques (also known as neuritic plaques, senile druse and brain druse) are extracellular deposits of amyloid beta in the grey matter of the brain." They cause diseases such as Alzheimer's disease, Parkinson's disease, Huntington's disease and play a role in most every other cognitive disorder due to the way this plaque gums of the neurons in your brain.

# With all this plaque caused by gluten,

# I have to wonder why this food

# hasn't been condemned yet?

## IF YOU LIKE BREAD,

## YOU'RE ADDICTION IS IN CONTROL OF YOU.

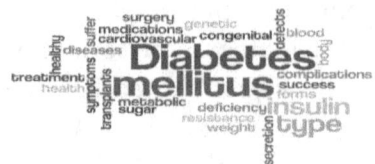

# UNLESS YOUR CHANGE YOUR EATING HABITS

# YOUR FATE IS WRITTEN IN THESE PAGES.

So, how do you stop the diabetes? It's actually a simple decision, stop eating foods that cause it, foods that contain wheat and grains. The problem is, following through on this decision, may be the hardest thing you'll ever have to achieve, because it involves breaking an addiction. The only solace you can take, is that you're not the only one and it's not your fault.

Nobody except a few doctors have come out and said what causes diabetes, I'm not a doctor, but I can tell you with full confidence what causes diabetes. It's the consumption of starchy carbohydrates.

Although it is possible to slow the progression of any of the diseases and disorders caused by diabetes, you cannot stop it without curbing the flow of glucose into the system completely and the only way to do that is to curb the carbs creating the glucose, as completely as possible.

We as a population have to do something to correct this aberration to our diet. This food is killing us painfully, expensively, indiscriminately and without dignity. As a society, we can't allow this to continue unabated, as it has, for the last 60 years. We must learn to "just say no" to glucose. The biggest problem is, the worse your addiction is the harder it is to break the addiction, but also the more important it is to break it. This could be the worst concern with carbohydrate addiction, there are different degrees of addiction, unlike that of heroin, cocaine and alcohol.

This problem manifests itself when trying to cut back as the greater your addiction is, the harder it will be to eliminate this food from your diet. But, it's essential that you eliminate it, because if you don't, the world of hurt described on *Carbs, The Newly Found Death Sentence*, will follow you until you either die or quit eating it. The easiest path to this goal is explained in *Carbs, How To Cut Back*

# Article 5
# Carbs and dementia

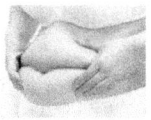

It's well documented how much of a pandemic obesity has become, worldwide. It's becoming evident that this pandemic of obesity is leading us into a pandemic of dementia, because obesity leads directly to dementia.

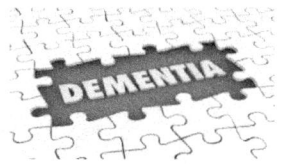

**Dementia is, after all, type 3 diabetes.**

If you're type 2 diabetic now and you don't change your eating habits, you stand a 100% chance of becoming type 3 diabetic. I can say this confidently because you don't have to be type 2 diabetic, to get type 3 diabetes, dementia. This is shown in the number of Alzheimer's patients now. That population is growing exponentially while the diabetic population just multiplies in numbers. Type2 diabetes just has a tendency to hasten the arrival of type3 diabetes.

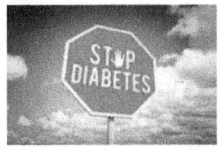

If we're to going stop this epidemic of dementia that's starting to cripple our population. We need to take drastic measures and the sooner we do so, the better our chance of survival. We have to slow the progression, where it starts, in what we eat. Thus, the reason for this article.

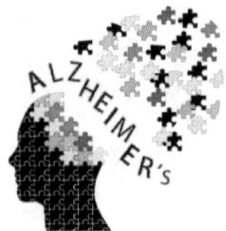 In most cases type 3 diabetes manifests itself in the disorder of Alzheimer's disease. I know that not everyone who has Alzheimer's disease has had type 2 diabetes, yet everyone who is type 2 diabetic will lose brain function. That science can't be changed. The only thing that can stop that runaway train is to stop feeding it. You must stop feeding carbohydrates into the fat factory that's responsible for it. Carbs are the only thing that can generate fat inside your body. It's this body fat, where the visceral fat lies that generates all the hormones and adipokines that dictate what this fat is going to do to your body. And it does plenty, all in the form of damage, damage to every system in your body as well as your brain. The more fat you have, the more damage it does to both.

The very first thing this fat does is to generate more fat through the use of the hormones that it produces, mainly leptin, along with Apelin and Chemerin, and it uses 100's of other adipokines to wreak havoc throughout your entire body, including your brain. These hormones block receptors in the brain that influence your behavior. This forces you to continue to feed fuel to the cycle unknowingly. I call this your fat factory. This is also called addiction and this is how the addiction of the fat factory works.

By blocking receptor neurons in the brain, the neuropeptides that signal your body, you're full and need to stop eating, can't do their job and tell you to stop eating. This is truly being controlled by your hormones. The pity of this cycle is, the larger you are, the more you experience it. It's a cycle that feeds itself and it's a science you can't change, without turning off the spigot.

It seems that this fat has become a self feeding disease, of its own. I've noticed that the worse you have the disease, the harder it is to kick. But it's also even more crucial to kick at that point, because it's already at the point of no return. Unless drastic measures are taken, a life of forgetfulness and lost memories is right around the corner, if it isn't happening already? When was the last time you lost your keys or couldn't remember someone's name?

Even though obesity is considered to be a disease by many, fat is considered by many professionals to be another internal organ. If so, it's one of the few organs that can grow in size, and when it does, it just multiplies the hormones' and adipokines' effects on our bodies exponentially, which isn't pretty.

Dictionary.com defines an organ as; "Biology a grouping of tissues into a distinct structure, as a heart or kidney in animals or a leaf or stamen in plants, that performs a specialized task."

By strict definition, fat follows that description. It is a group of tissues in a distinct structure, that performs a specialized task. In this case it performs many tasks, so many that it's mind boggling. This one organ can create more cytokines and hormones than any other organ in the body. That means that fat is one organ in our bodies, that either controls us, or we control it. When I talk about controlling us, I'm talking about control of our hormones which in turn controls our emotions. It also means that this one organ is responsible for more illness and disease than anything else in our entire bodies.

This is exactly why it's so bad - the worst of these adipokines are cell signaling proteins that trigger hosts of illnesses and diseases. These diseases range from multiple cancers to multiple CVDs, which we'll talk about later. The fat creates the bad cytokines that muck up your system. They create the adipokines that instruct your cells to turn into amyloid plaque. Amyloids are the foundation of an arm long list of disorders, many cancers including breast cancer, colorectal cancer, stomach cancer, pancreatic cancer, liver cancer, and on and on. This isn't even mentioning the mental disorders that come with amyloids. That list is even longer. The devastating effects that these hormones and adipokines have on your body, because of the fat in your body, are truly astounding.

I can see now that glucose not only creates fat, the fat it creates, creates in turn, hormones and adipokines that trigger the inflammation and cell degradation associated with cancer and CVDs and worst of all, brain loss. This fat factory that is feeding itself by turning our hormones against us, is wasting away our brains and taking with it, all of our mental faculties and what's left of our dignity.

But it's not only the fat factory that's destroying our brains. It's the gliadin that you eat every time you eat gluten. Your body can have this auto-immune

41

response to gliadin, by sending out anti-gliadin antibodies that have the ability to attach themselves to purkinje cells in your cerebellum as explained by Dr Davis;. "The antigliadin antibodies triggered by gluten can bind to Purkinje cells of the brain, cells unique to the cerebellum. Brain tissue such as Purkinje cells do not have the capacity to regenerate: Once damaged, cerebellar Purkinje cells are gone . . . forever." Doesn't that say brain damage?

Only by taking abrupt action immediately, are you going to interrupt the production of the anti-gliadin antibodies eating up your brain and the hormones that the fat factory is producing. And it's producing these hormones so it can continue to enlarge itself in a vicious cycle. The only way to stop this cycle at this point, is to stop the fuel that feeds it, carbohydrates.

I'm sorry, but there's no way around it. Not even you can change science. Unless you shut off the spigot of inflammation that you're pouring into your body, every time you eat carbs, you're going to feed the fat that feeds the inflammation that causes all the disorders and disease listed in *Carbs, The New Death Sentence.* (When I say that I'm sorry, I mean it. I used to be addicted to them and I know what it takes to break their grip of addiction.)

A search of *Obesity and brain size* at NIH's PMC site brought up over 1200 studies done on obesity and brain size. One in particular that I looked at, showed the influence leptin has on the brain and its ability to regulate energy in the body. Leptin is one of hundreds of hormones and adipokines (cell signaling proteins), that's manufactured in your body fat.

According to a study on Obesity and Dementia; "Within the brain, leptin regulates energy intake" "Leptin inhibits the expression of orexigenic neuropeptides and stimulates the expression of anorexigenic neuropeptides, which results in inhibition of energy intake (*Jequier, 2002*)."

That explains why those on a diet high in carbs (which is the only thing that can make people fat), run out of energy so often and need to refuel every two hours or so. It's the leptin expressing itself in the brain, that inhibits the signals, that tell you if you have enough energy or not and if you need to eat or not. And this is where the problem multiplies. Since leptin is formed in the fat around your body, it tells your brain that your body needs more fat by blocking these signals. So what do you do? You eat more, to feed that need. This is leptin resistance, the leptin blocking those receptors in your brain that tell you that you don't need to eat and have enough energy.

If you don't have the ability to fight your hormones (leptin in this case) and resist this basic expression of survival, hunger, you're doomed to everything listed in *Carbs, The New Death Sentence*. That is what makes carbs so addictive and dangerous and why their continuance must be curbed.

"It is known that adipokines, secretory products of adipose tissue such as leptin, interact directly with specific nuclei in certain areas of the brain such as the hippocampus. This results in regulation of not only feeding behavior, but also neurodegeneration, synaptic plasticity, neurogenesis and memory consolidation (*Doherty, 2011*)."

According to another study on Obesity, leptin and Dementia; "Amyloid fibril formation is considered to be a signature of neurodegenerative processes. The exact processes leading to cellular degeneration remain unknown although several amyloid-involving mechanisms have been proposed. Amyloids occupy the extracellular space and destroy the structure of cells and tissues, amyloid fibrils destabilize cell membranes, Some proteins forming amyloids, for instance α-synuclein which contributes to the formation of intracellular Lewy bodies in Parkinson's disease, other proteins with an unordered structure are the IAPP in type II diabetes and β-amyloid in Alzheimer's disease . Such an unfolded structure allows the protein to be rather easily self-assembled into fibrils."

The first adipokine, leptin was discovered in 1994 and since then 100's have been discovered. Isn't that disturbing? Fat that we make from glucose manufacturers hosts of hormones that are wreaking havoc on our bodies.

That means, with the carbs you eat, you're making fat, a fat that grows hormones that are cell signaling proteins that control hunger, energy expenditure and fat oxidation, blood pressure, glucose uptake and insulin resistance just to begin with. I didn't even make it half way through all the cell signaling proteins that were listed. The others that I did check all triggered a disorder or inflammation somewhere in the body. Many of them are associated with more than half of the known cancers, a multitude of heart diseases and every form of dementia known to man.

Leptin only plays a small part in the assault that our hormones throw at us. Adiponectin plays just as important role. As does Apelin, chemerin, and 6 other hormones that they've found so far. And they're finding more. All these hormones are adipokines and are manufactured in adipose tissue or fat. The other six adipokines listed on Wikipedia that I didn't list here are all associated with inflammation and the oxidative stress that's associated with almost all cancers, most heart diseases and all brain damage that's not caused by concussions and blunt force trauma.

If leptin plays a part in neurodegeneration, synaptic plasticity, neurogenesis and memory consolidation, doesn't it make sense that it's the creation of leptin that we need to control, to stem its influence in our bodies? If we're to control the amount of leptin in our bodies, and leptin is made in adipose tissue (fat), then we need to control the amount of fat in our bodies. The only thing that controls the amount of fat that goes into our bodies is the amount of glucose that we feed it. We know that the glucose is controlled by the amount of carbs we put in our bodies.

You can't change the science. Glucose in the body creates fat. Fat creates leptin. The more leptin you have in your body, the more resistant you become to it and the more it needs to feed itself. It's a cycle that keeps feeding itself again and again and again until you're hungry 10 minutes right after you finished a big meal. I can remember times after a big spaghetti dinner when I was foraging though the cabinets and refrigerator, looking for something else to eat, on a full stomach.

When I think about that now, I think, how sick could I have been to be expressing that kind of behavior? Then I think, I was a kid then, I was only eating what was fed to me. Here's the scary part, I was eating exactly what the ADA was telling me I should eat. That's exactly what you're doing right now, following the dietary guidelines that you grew up with. How could they have gotten it so wrong?

Fortunately. I can only remember those times now, as I don't get hungry much anymore. (Another advantage of being thin, and on a ketogenic diet.) Leptin doesn't control anything in my body. I don't have that much leptin in my body to control my urges and my energy. With a body fat ratio of 17 %, my body isn't ever going to make enough leptin to create any problems in my body, provided that I don't feed it what it wants, carbohydrates. This is what make it so easy now, to fast.

This is where Adiponectin plays its role. "Adiponectin is a protein hormone that modulates a number of metabolic processes, including glucose regulation and fatty acid oxidation." It's adiponectin that not only dictates how glucose is turned into fat, it controls how the fat is burned in the body, and this is where it gets real interesting. Higher levels of adiponectin in the body allow the body to generate more energy from a smaller amount of fat, making adiponectin crucial for maximum energy output with minimal intake of food. That is why Dr Miller says that "people on low carb, diets have more energy."

Since adiponectin is made in adipose tissue like all other adipokines, one would think that having a lot of fat would create a lot of adiponectin, when actually, we create just as much of it if not more when we don't have the fat stores in our bodies. Our bodies use fat in our bones to create adiponectin. Actually, "Levels of the hormone are inversely correlated with body fat percentage in adults" "Contrary to expectations, despite being produced in adipose tissue, adiponectin was found to be decreased in obesity. "

"The hormone plays a role in the suppression of the metabolic derangements that may result in type 2 diabetes, obesity, atherosclerosis, non-alcoholic fatty liver disease (NAFLD) and an independent risk factor for metabolic syndrome."

So, how do we increase this hormone? Since levels of the hormone are inversely correlated with body fat percentage, the more fat we have, the less adiponectin we have in our systems. This in itself, leads to more obesity, more diabetes and everything that comes along with that.

Again According to Wikipedia; "Weight reduction significantly increases circulating levels. A low level of adiponectin is an *independent* risk factor for developing: Metabolic syndrome and Diabetes mellitus "

That means to avoid low levels of adiponectin in your body, weight loss is crucial. This places more importance in calorie restriction and fasting. But there's good news for those carboholics who have trouble restricting their calories, "...omega-3 fatty acids eicosapentaenoic acid (EPA) and docosahexaenoic acid (DHA) have shown increased plasma adiponectin. Curcumin, capsaicin, gingerol, and catechins have also been found to increase adiponectin expression. "

Fasting brings other benefits with it as well, as it's important to the health of your brain. It not only boosts brain growth, it boosts anti-oxidant production which keeps you healthier by being better able to fight off illness and disease. Fasting conjures up images of starvation with it, though. This may be true is you are one of those unfortunate individuals who is still stuck on a carbohydrate diet. On a carbohydrate diet, fasting is next to impossible. At the least, it's very difficult and involves a massive amount of discomfort.

**The best way to avoid this is to convert your diet to a low carb diet, preferably a diet without any carbs.**

How do we discourage the consumption of these foods, without upsetting the giant food industrial complex? We can't. It's their responsibility that Americans are in this predicament. It's their advertising that's driven this massive consumption of carbs that is creating all the disease this food is responsible for.

I wonder what would happen if you taxed carbohydrates by the amount of fat they create, which is influenced directly by their place on the glycemic index? Would this force the population to cut back on their intake of this dangerous food? It will definitely help to pay for all the medical needs that carboholics are going to need, if they continue to consume these killing field grains.

# Article 6

## Carbs and Cancer Go Together Like Beetle & Juice

Cancer is responsible for over 8,200,000 deaths every year. Playing a major influence in half of the different types of cancer, listed below, is one common thread that permeates our diets everywhere, carbohydrates or wheat, sugar and grain based foods. This one basic staple that we're all encouraged to eat massive quantities of, is actually what's killing us. The worst aspect of this whole problem is that we were told to eat it. We were told that it should be the largest portion of our meals and that we eat it on a daily basis. We were told to do this because, it was thought, that it was healthy for us.

**I mentioned in Carbs! The Newly Discovered Death Sentence,**

**this is not healthy food, I intend to prove it in this article.**

Because of the lack of studies done of the effects of wheat in the diet and cancer, it's not always easy to piece the information together. Many of the studies that were done years ago have been suppressed from public knowledge and are not easy to obtain now. Dr Davis and Dr Perlmutter have already located many of these studies and they can be found in their books, *Wheat Belly* and *Grain Brain*. I spent only enough time to decipher sugar and wheat's influence in half of the various types of cancer listed below. If the Consumer Protection Safety Council is considering warnings for chemicals that cause cancer, (which they are in California) why isn't anyone considering warnings for the consumption of these food staples, sugar and flour?

Suffice it to say, there is enough evidence here to prove that this food source should come with the same warning that everything that causes cancer has to bear, like cigarettes, and now, processed meats and fast foods, and chemicals in California. (California's attorney general, Bill

47

Lockyer, filed suit in August against McDonald's; Burger King; Frito-Lay, owned by PepsiCo; and six other food companies, saying that they should be forced to put labels on all fries and potato chips sold in California. The proposed warning might say something to this effect: *"This product contains a chemical known to the state of California to cause cancer."*

It's interesting that California is going after fast food companies for the "cancer causing French fries" when it's the bread that has as much if not more influence on cancer as trans-fats. I'll admit, French fries play a definite role in cancer, but if they'd only look at the real reason that they cause cancer, it's due to their influence on your blood glucose and this is exactly how sugar and wheat are responsible for cancer, diabetes, HBP, cardio-vascular disease, digestive disorders, etc. If they concentrated on the glucose side of the equation, they'd soon have labels on everything that flour and sugar are used in. This article is going to show how this food actually contributes to the environmental factors that are at the root cause of many cancers. (Environmental factor in this case is glucose or sugar from your diet and lifestyle.)

**Cancer** - a large family of known diseases that affect humans. causing 8.2 million deaths as of 2012 The great majority of cancers, some 90–95% of cases, are due to environmental factors. The remaining 5–10% are due to inherited genetics. Environmental, as used by cancer researchers, means any cause that is not inherited genetically, such as lifestyle, economic and behavioral factors, and not merely pollution. Common environmental factors that contribute to cancer death include tobacco (25–30%), diet and obesity (30–35%), infections (15–20%), radiation (both ionizing and non-ionizing, up to 10%), stress, lack of physical activity, and environmental pollutants. Diet, physical inactivity, and obesity are related to up to 30–35% of cancer deaths.

## THE LARGEST INFLUENCE IN OBESITY IS CARBOHYDRATES THE CARBS YOU FIND IN WHEAT, SUGAR AND ALL GRAIN BASED FOODS.

We only have time to look at a few of the hundreds of different kinds of cancer. Of the 12 listed below, we'll look at 6 of those in detail further below:

1. **Lung cancer** - 1.56 million **deaths annually**, as of 2012

2. **Pancreatic cancer** - 330,000 **deaths** globally

3. **Colorectal (colon) cancer** – 610,000 deaths
   (Inflammatory bowel disease - 51,000 **deaths** in 2013 due to inflammatory bowel disease (largest influence to colorectal cancer) alone.)

4. **Breast cancer** - 18.2% of all cancer deaths for men and women together or 283,920 deaths

5. **Liver cancer** - In 2013, 300,000 deaths from liver cancer were due to hepatitis B, hepatitis C, or alcohol

6. **Thyroid cancer** - in 2010, 36,000 deaths globally up from 24,000 in 1990. Obesity may be associated with a higher incidence of thyroid cancer, but this relationship remains the subject of much debate.

7. **Ovarian cancer** - estimated 15,000 deaths in 2008

8. **Cervical cancer** - 266,000 deaths

9. **Prostate Cancer** - In 2010 it resulted in 256,000 deaths up from 156,000 deaths in 1990.

10. **Bladder cancer** - is the 9th leading cause of cancer with 430,000 new cases

11. **Kidney cancer** -17,870 deaths in the US and the UK alone in 2012, with 208,000 new cases each year

12. **Endometrial cancer** - caused 76,000 deaths


**Let's take a closer look at some of these types of cancer;**

**Lung cancer** - 1.56 million deaths worldwide, annually as of 2012, is the most common cause of cancer in the US. The most common cause of lung cancer is smoking which requires warnings on all cigarette packs. The only link carbs have to lung cancer, is that they control your emotions through controlling your hormones. This would control you in its influence when you're hungry, and instead of eating, opt for a cigarette instead. How many people trying to quit smoking end up putting on weight?

**Breast cancer** - 18.2% of all cancer deaths for men and women together or 283,920 deaths is the second most common cause of cancer related deaths in women. The largest risk factors are obesity, lack of physical exercise, hormone replacement therapy during menopause, drinking alcohol, ionizing radiation, early age menstruation, having children late or not at all, older age, and family history. Dietary iodine deficiency may also play a role. There is a definite relationship between diet and breast cancer, including an increased risk with a high fat diet, alcohol intake, and obesity, related to higher cholesterol levels. Don't forget, that nothing builds fat and cholesterol in the system more than starchy carbohydrates, wheat, sugar and grains. "High cholesterol levels" here, are what's used to refer to high LDL levels, as high HDL levels are beneficial. High LDL levels, as you'll see in article 11, are the beneficiary of a high carbohydrate diet. What would happen to breast cancer if you removed wheat, sugar and grains from the diet? Would that put a hamper of the spread of cancer? I've never seen a warning, that obesity can cause breast cancer, or that eating grain based foods can cause obesity.

**Prostate Cancer** - In 2010 it resulted in 256,000 deaths up from 156,000 deaths in 1990 and is the leading cause of cancer death in males worldwide. The data on the relationship between diet and prostate cancer is poor. In light of this the rate of prostate cancer is linked to the consumption of the Western diet. There is little if any evidence to support an association between trans fat, saturated fat and carbohydrate intake and risk of prostate cancer. Evidence regarding the role of omega-3 fatty acids in preventing prostate cancer does not suggest that they reduce the risk of prostate cancer, although additional research is needed. Vitamin supplements appear to have no effect and some may increase the risk. High calcium intake has been linked to advanced prostate cancer. Consuming fish may lower prostate cancer deaths but does not appear to affect its occurrence. Some evidence supports lower rates of prostate cancer with a vegetarian diet. There is some tentative evidence for foods containing lycopene and selenium. Diets rich in cruciferous vegetables, soy, beans and other legumes may be associated with a lower risk of prostate cancer, especially more advanced cancers. Men who get regular exercise may have a slightly lower risk, especially vigorous activity and the risk of advanced prostate cancer. "Diets rich in cruciferous vegetables" tells me that "cole crops", leafy green vegetables like cabbage, Brussels sprouts, kale and broccoli, foods that are high in fiber are key to not upsetting the glucose levels in the blood, as well as providing the micronutrients necessary for resistance. Maintaining low glucose levels in the blood seems to be crucial to avoiding prostate disease. The more fiber a food has, the slower it releases its glucose.

**Colorectal cancer** – 610,000 deaths-Inflammatory bowel disease - 51,000 deaths in 2013, is the largest influence to colorectal cancer. Colon cancer is a complex disease which arises as a result of the interaction of environmental and genetic factors. It is increasingly thought that alterations to enteral (probiotics?) bacteria can contribute to inflammatory gut diseases, which has the largest influence on IBD. IBD affected individuals have been found to have 30-50 percent reduced biodiversity of commensalism bacteria such as a decrease in Firmicutes (namely lachnosperacieae and Bacteroidetes), what I believe are probiotics (but I can't find a definitive answer to that). Further evidence of the role of gut flora in the cause of inflammatory bowel disease is that IBD affected individuals are more likely to have been prescribed antibiotics in the 2-5 year period before their diagnosis than unaffected individuals. The enteral bacteria can be altered by environmental factors, such as concentrated milk fats (a common ingredient of processed foods and confectionery) or oral medications such as antibiotics and oral iron preparations. This tells me that those who are taking headache medication (NSAIDs) often, are themselves open for colorectal cancer and one thing we know about wheat and grain consumption is that it causes headaches, forcing one to use NSAIDs for pain relief.

**Liver cancer** - In 2013, 300,000 deaths from liver cancer were due to hepatitis B, hepatitis C, or alcohol. Liver cancer, also known as hepatic cancer, is a cancer that originates in the liver. The leading cause of liver cancer is cirrhosis due to either hepatitis B, hepatitis C, or alcohol. Cirrhosis is most commonly caused by alcohol, hepatitis B, hepatitis C, and non-alcoholic fatty liver disease. Non-alcoholic fatty liver disease (NAFLD) is one of the causes of fatty liver (a contributor to liver cancer); occurring when fat is deposited (steatosis) in the liver due to causes other than excessive alcohol use. NAFLD is related to insulin resistance and the metabolic syndrome and may respond to treatments originally developed for other insulin-resistant states (e.g.diabetes mellitus type 2) such as weight loss. We know that carbohydrate consumption in the form of wheat and grains cause insulin resistance. Doesn't it make sense then, that the consumption of wheat and grains play a major influence in liver cancer?

**Kidney cancer** - Factors that increase the risk of kidney cancer include smoking, which can double the risk of the disease; regular use of NSAIDs such as ibuprofen and naproxen, which may increase the risk by 51% ; obesity; faulty genes; a family history of kidney cancer; having kidney disease that needs dialysis; being infected with hepatitis C; and previous treatment for testicular cancer or cervical cancer. There are also other possible risk factors such as kidney stones and high blood pressure, which are being investigated. 17,870 deaths in the US and the UK alone in 2012, with 208,000 new cases each year. Again, obesity and the use of NSAIDs for headaches, show the dangers of carbohydrate consumption.

**Bladder cancer** – is the 9th leading cause of cancer with 430,000 new cases and 165,000 deaths occurring in 2012. Urothelial carcinoma is a prototypical example of a malignancy arising from environmental carcinogenic influences. By far the important cause is cigarette smoking, which contributes to approximately half of the disease burden. Chemical exposures such as those sustained by workers in the petroleum industry, the manufacture of paints and pigments (prototypically aniline dyes), and agrochemicals are known to predispose to urothelial cancer. This is the one factor that intrigues me the most, the influence of agrochemicals in the disease. Some of the most treated foods in our diet are wheat, corn, soy and grain based foods. They genetically modify these foods to withstand the rigors of agrochemicals like herbicides and insecticides, both of which contribute to bladder cancer. What is the one food that we were all told to eat the most of? Grains. If this one food were taken out of the diet, would that affect the numbers of people dying from bladder cancer? I think so. (I'm sure Monsanto, Syngenta and Bayer won't.)

**Pancreatic cancer** - 330,000 deaths globally each year. Risk factors for pancreatic adenocarcinoma include:

1.  Age, gender, and race; the risk of developing pancreatic cancer increases with age. Most cases occur after age 65, while cases before age 40 are uncommon. The disease is slightly more common in men than women, and in the United States is over 1.5 times more common in African Americans, though incidence in Africa is low. The explanation for this was given in the foreword. African Americans as a race, have not had the time to adapt their physiology to handle the influx of glucose that carbs put into the system.

2.  Cigarette smoking is the well-established avoidable risk factor for pancreatic cancer by many researchers, approximately doubling risk among long-term smokers, the risk increasing with the number of

cigarettes smoked and the years of smoking. Apparently the "best established risk factor" according to the scientific community is not what the next three reasons involve, probably due to their inability to see through their own addiction making them unaware of the influence that glucose has on pancreatic function. With a 280% greater chance of pancreatic cancer due to having type 2 diabetes, I'm surprised that they don't recognize the most avoidable risk factor as being excess glucose in the blood, requiring a greater need for insulin.

3. Chronic pancreatitis appears to almost triple risk, and as with diabetes, new-onset pancreatitis may be a symptom of a tumor. The risk of pancreatic cancer in individuals with familial pancreatitis is particularly high.

4. Diabetes mellitus is a risk factor for pancreatic cancer. People who have been diagnosed with Type 2 diabetes for longer than ten years may have a 50% increased risk, as compared with non-diabetics.

5. Obesity; a BMI greater than 35 increases relative risk by about half. Family history; 5–10% of pancreatic cancer cases have an inherited component, where people have a family history of pancreatic cancer.

6. High level of triglycerides in the blood.

It appears to me that the most common cause of Pancreatic cancer deals with **ECC,** excessive carbohydrate consumption or excess glucose in the system, is not hard to understand at all, considering this person is under the same spell that everyone else is under....your addiction to carbohydrates. Because of his addiction, this person is unable to see its influence in these cancers. Because of this, the only reasons they can only look at, are ones that don't include their addiction. Lose the addiction, lose the cancers.

If 90 – 95% of all cases of cancer are due to lifestyle and behavioral factors, what does that say about our eating habits? Our eating habits are the most influential factor in anyone's lifestyle. The old adage, "you are what you eat", is more valid here, than anywhere else. Our individual diets are what separate us from each other more than almost anything else, as that's what distinguishes us from each other. In every diet, there exists one common thread throughout the world, and that's grains, wheat in the western hemisphere and rice in the eastern hemisphere. They're in every diet of every ethnicity. This is the one common thread that affects everyone on the planet. It does so simply because it's in every diet on the planet, in some fashion or another.

As evidenced above, there are at least 6 types of cancer in this article, alone, in which wheat and grains play a part. If you eat foods that cause cancer, you'll more than likely, contract cancer. What if this one factor was removed from the equation of cancer? What if wheat and grains were removed from our diets? What would happen if you took that one factor in the equation of cancer, out of the equation? Would you still come still come up with the same result?

I contend that it would change the whole equation enough that the end result of cancer would inevitably be changed. This begs the question, if we removed wheat and grains from the diet, would that be a start for a cure for many of these cancers? I understand why a warning label is on every pack of cigarettes, one should be, we know that smoking causes lung cancer. If they put out warnings for something that may cause cancer, like processed meats and 'fast foods', why can't they put out a warning for something that clearly causes cancer.... sugar and wheat based products?

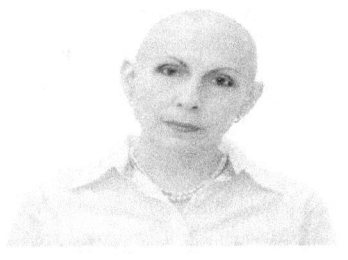

# Article 7
## CARBS AND HIGH BLOOD PRESSURE

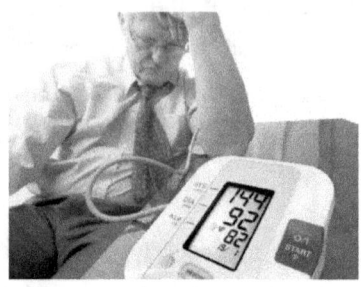

This is something that I don't even like to talk about because I have high blood pressure. Even though I control it now, because I had high blood pressure in the past, my doctor says that I have high blood pressure now. But she went on to say that I control my high blood pressure, now. I guess that's true, but I won't control my blood pressure with medication. I refuse to. I control mine with diet.

The last three times I saw the doctor, for the first time in my life that I can remember, my blood pressure was as perfect as you could get, 120/60. It was always something around 145/90, 168/95 or what it usually was at rest, 132/86. I can remember a nurse checking my blood pressure after waking up from spending a month in coma. My blood pressure at that time was 132/86. I thought that was normal. I didn't learn until recently that it was actually elevated. Even though it wasn't considered that elevated at the time, it's been recently learned that elevation even in this small amount, does enough damage to internal organs that it puts undue strain on the heart, to have to pump harder to get all the blood it needs to, to fuel your entire body.

Hypertension usually does not cause symptoms initially, but sustained hypertension over time is a major risk factor for hypertensive heart disease, coronary artery disease, stroke, aortic aneurysm, peripheral artery disease, *and* chronic kidney disease.

I can tell you what it's like to have a stroke. They're no fun. I still live with the residual effects from the stroke that I had 31 years ago, hemiplegia (right side paralysis). I'm partially paralyzed today from a massive stroke that I had from a severe closed head injury, 31 years ago. I know very well what it's like to suffer a massive stroke. To say the very least, it is life changing.

Of the two types of hypertension, primary and secondary, 90% - 95% are primary. They are defined *"with no natural cause"*, yet I've learned the real cause. Secondary hypertension is always the result of a chronic disease or disorder, such as narrowing of the aorta or arteries or kidney disease (narrowing of the kidney arteries). Endocrine disorders such as excess aldosterone, cortisol, or catecholamines have also been known to be responsible for secondary hypertension.

I've learned that dietary changes lower blood pressure better than any medication. The best part of that is that I don't have to worry about buying my medication or remembering to take it. Simple dietary changes are enough to guarantee that I won't have to deal with hypertension or any of its consequences, hypertensive heart disease

Essential hypertension (also called primary hypertension or idiopathic hypertension) is the form of hypertension that according to the National Heart Association has no identifiable cause. It is the most common type of hypertension, affecting 95% of hypertensive patients. It tends to be familial and is likely to be the consequence of an interaction between environmental and genetic factors. The prevalence of essential hypertension increases with *age*, and individuals with relatively high blood pressure at younger ages are at increased risk for the subsequent development of hypertension. Hypertension can increase the risk of cerebral, cardiac, and renal events.

I define them as caused by carbs because I know the value of restricting carbs in my diet and what that did to control my blood pressure. I attribute my first and continued experience with normal blood pressure to my diet that contains no high starchy carbohydrates in it. Glucose, sugar, carbs, the food that kills, does more so, by causing hypertension, the precursor to most cardiovascular diseases and disorders.

It's interesting that the most common type of hypertension, tends to be familial and is likely to be the consequence of an interaction between environmental and genetic factors.

The most important of those environmental and genetic factors, happens to be diet. The one thing that never changes in a family's diet that's passed down from generation to generation, is the amount of carbohydrates in the diet. What's changed over time, is the carbohydrate itself. It's become less nutritious. It's become more dangerous because it creates more dirty LDL particles in the blood, which in turn creates more plaque clogging the arteries, raising the blood pressure.

Hypertension is one of the most common disorders affecting almost every other disorder. By definition, essential hypertension has no identifiable cause. However, several *risk factors* have been identified. Most authoritative voices claim that there is no identifiable cause for essential hypertension. Most of these voices aren't aware of how carbs influence inflammation in the blood and how that influences HBP.

The reason they see *"no identifiable cause"*, apparently is because nobody wants to consider, that the carbs that cause glycation could be the cause for HBP, probably because they are just as addicted to them as everyone else. I know for certain that the major contributing factor for essential hypertension is glucose. Anyone who's on the diet that I'm on (ketogenic), can tell you the very same thing, especially if they suffered from hypertension in the past.

**Carbs are the major contributing factor for hypertension.**

*"One possible mechanism involves a reduction in vascular compliance due to the stiffening of the arteries."* This is what interests me. If a reduction in vascular compliance due to stiffening of the arteries is a possible mechanism, we should look at what causes this reduction in vascular compliance. Since it's due to stiffening of the arteries, we need to look at what stiffens the arteries, Atheroma or atheromatous plaque, a buildup of deposits within the wall of an artery.

*Veins* cannot not develop atheromata, unless surgically moved to function as an artery, as in bypass surgery. This disease is the product of apoB LDL particles glycating and leaving atheroma plaque residue which in turn deposits itself in your arteries. While the early stages, based on gross appearance, have traditionally been termed *fatty streaks* by pathologists, they are not composed of fat cells, i.e. *adipose cells*, but of accumulations of *white blood cells*, especially *macrophages*, that have taken up oxidized *low-density lipoprotein* (LDL). After they accumulate large amounts of cytoplasmic membranes (with associated high cholesterol content) they are called foam cells. When foam cells die, their contents are released, which attracts more macrophages and creates an extracellular lipid core near the center to inner surface of each atherosclerotic plaque. Conversely, the outer, older portions of the plaque become more calcified, less metabolically active and more physically stiff over time.

This is evidence to me that what stiffens the arteries is carried in the LDL particles simply because those are the particles that feed the cells. A backup of these LDL particles occurs when your HDL particles are too low to remove the spent fuel from the LDL particles. It's this back up of LDL particles, that leads to the massive glycation that leads to the spread of plaque and cytokines throughout your entire body. This is also the start of inflammation.

In short, it's glycation of the LDL cholesterol that deposits foam cells in the tunica intima of the artery. That is what stiffens the artery and restricts blood flow increasing blood pressure. Understand what creates LDL particles in the body by reading *The Value of Balancing Your Cholesterol* or *The Foundation of LDL Cholesterol*. They explain exactly how carbs are the major influence of dirty LDL cholesterol in the body.

Reduce the "dirty" LDL cholesterol and you'll reduce the amount of plaque that flows through your system, which in turn will guard against stiffening your arteries and raising your blood pressure. Restrict the carbs and you'll reduce the dirty LDL cholesterol, limiting hypertension. Again, can it be that simple? Maybe not easy, but a simple solution to controlling hypertension is to curb your carb consumption to control your weight. For me, nothing worked better.

Obesity has shown to increase the risk of high blood pressure fivefold, as compared to normal weight. As many as two-thirds of hypertension cases can be attributed to being overweight with over 85% of cases occurring with a body mass index over 25. Obesity was shown to be a definitive link in all hypertensive cases. A definitive link between obesity and hypertension has been found using animal and clinical studies; from these it has been realized that many mechanisms are potential causes of obesity-induced hypertension. These mechanisms include the activation of the sympathetic nervous system as well as the activation of the renin–angiotensin-aldosterone system." Obviously, this author is completely unaware of how carbohydrates contribute to hypertension, probably due to his own addiction.

That makes me wonder, does diabetes also contribute to hypertension? "Hypertension can also be caused by Insulin resistance and/or hyperinsulinemia, which are components of syndrome X, or the metabolic syndrome." Insulin is a polypeptide hormone secreted by cells in the islets of Langerhans, which are contained throughout the pancreas. By converting glucose to fat, its main purpose is to regulate the levels of glucose in the body antagonistically with glucagon through negative feedback loops. Insulin also exhibits vasodilatory properties. In normotensive individuals, insulin may stimulate sympathetic activity without elevating mean arterial pressure.

"Dietary and lifestyle changes to lower blood pressure and decrease the risk of health complications" seems to be the underlying theme in diminishing high blood pressure. When they talk about dietary changes, the issue here is weight, and the fact that most of you are carrying too much of it. We all know what influences weight more than anything else, starchy carbs. This is the reasoning behind my conclusion that carbs are the major cause of high blood pressure. Again like the cause of cancer, if you remove any ingredient that it takes to make something, you cannot make that thing anymore and if we remove carbs from the equation of hypertension, it changes the equation completely. If you can curb the carbs, you can cure the disorder,

Many people affected by hypertension are not labeled as hypertensive, therefore hypertension is a problem that may be better addressed by educating the entire population of its dangers and how it affects all other functions in the body. Because of the prevalence of hypertension, most doctors now advise on lifestyle changes prior to drug intervention.

The 2004 British Hypertension Society guidelines proposed the following lifestyle changes consistent with those outlined by the US National High BP Education Program in 2002 for the primary prevention of hypertension:

- maintain normal body weight for adults (e.g. body mass index 20–25 kg/m$^2$)
- reduce dietary sodium intake to <100 mmol/ day (<6 g of sodium chloride or <2.4 g of sodium per day)
- engage in regular aerobic physical activity such as brisk walking (≥30 min per day, most days of the week)
- limit alcohol consumption to no more than 3 units/day in men and no more than 2 units/day in women
- consume a diet rich in fruit and vegetables (e.g. at least five portions per day);

Effective lifestyle modification may lower blood pressure as much as an individual antihypertensive drug. Combinations of two or more lifestyle modifications can achieve even better results."

The first thing they mention is to maintain a normal body weight for adults. We all know that limiting carbohydrates is crucial to maintaining a normal body weight, hence, limiting carbohydrates are crucial to limiting hypertension. In my estimation, that means that carbs are a primary cause of hypertension. It makes sense that blood without excess, sticky glucose in it, will flow much easier  than blood that has massive amounts of this gooey, gluey, substance that comes from carbs, in it to clog things up. Is this another DUH?

"The first line of treatment for hypertension is lifestyle changes, including dietary changes, physical exercise, and weight loss. These have all been shown to significantly reduce blood pressure in people with hypertension. Their potential effectiveness is similar to and at times exceeds a single medication. If hypertension is high enough to justify immediate use of medications, lifestyle changes are still recommended in conjunction with medication."

Diet has taken the place of medication for me and it works better than the medication ever did. Lifestyle changes when it comes to obesity, refer to weight loss, but here the recommendations refer only to limiting the use of salt. My contention is that salt isn't that important if you limit the primary ingredients that are responsible, and that's the starchy carbs you get from all grain based foods, the foundation all dirty LDL cholesterol. Again, is this addiction speaking, keeping the author from seeing the truth?

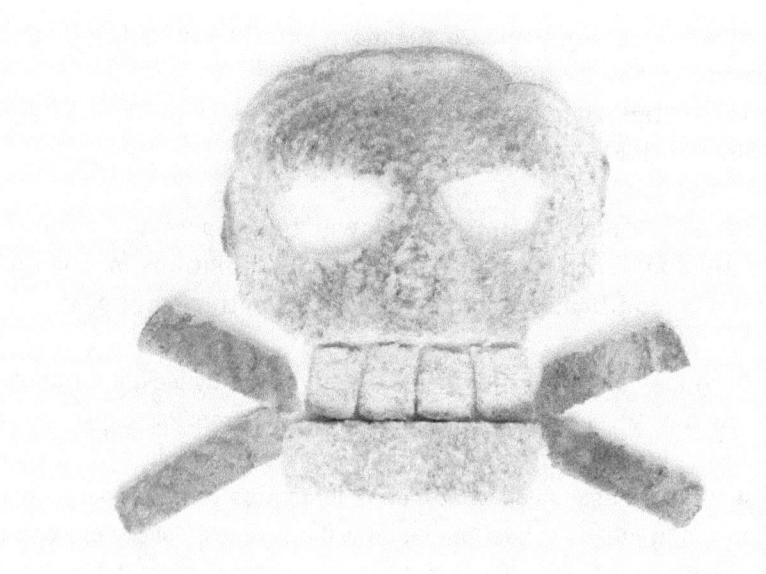

# IT'S TIME FOR YOUR CURE!

# IT BEGINS WITH YOUR DIET!

# THE BEST PART IS,

# IT'S FREE

# ARTICLE 8
# CARBS AND THEIR INFLUENCE IN
# HEART DISEASE

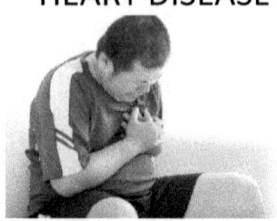

With the rise in cardiovascular diseases and the deaths occurring from it, it's a wonder that this major cause of them is still allowed to be advertised as much as it is. With over 17,300,000 deaths, worldwide, alone, in 2013, our society thinks it's more important to find new drugs to suppress the symptoms instead of finding a lasting cure, that doesn't include any drugs at all. I guess there's no money in it. That forces me to think, is that what society wants, or is that what their being sold?

Carbohydrate influence in many heart diseases is clearly undeniable. Whereas cancer is a catch all term, for a myriad of diseases, heart disease and cardiovascular diseases are catch-all phrases for all diseases involving the heart and circulatory system. That alone makes it difficult, to nail down any one agent, source or reason for its pervasiveness in these diseases. Yet, there is one common thread that shows up in at least half of these diseases – inflammation. Inflammation's largest contributor is glucose. Glucose's largest contributor is carbs. They're woven from two strands, sugar and flour - grain based products from wheat (gluten),corn, rice and oats in particular. This article is going to look at carbs influence on as many cardiovascular diseases as we can and I'm going to talk about carbs influence, in each one, again showing just how dangerous these food staples (flour and sugar) are. (Of course when I mention flour, I'm talking about all wheat and grain products, because the two most prevalent, wheat and corn, are ground into flour before their preparation, to make into foods, before marketing.) It's this grinding into flour that takes away any fiber that the food ever had. Flour and water make paste which is so quick to digest and break down to its basic form, glucose, that it loses any nutrition that it ever held. To get a better idea of the scope of cardiovascular diseases and the role carbs play in each one, I'll list as many of them as I can, and attempt to tie each disease to what influences it most. There are many cardiovascular diseases involving the blood vessels. They are known as vascular diseases as well as cardiovascular diseases.

Vascular diseases include:

1.  Coronary artery disease(also known as coronary heart disease and ischemic heart disease)
2.  Peripheral arterial disease– disease of blood vessels that supply blood to the arms and legs
3.  Cerebrovascular disease– disease of blood vessels that supply blood to the brain (includes stroke)
4.  Renal artery stenosis
5.  Aortic aneurysm

There are also many cardiovascular diseases that involve the heart and since all vascular diseases deal with plaque in the arterial walls, we're going to be looking at the ones that deal with the heart itself; Together they resulted in 17.3 million deaths (31.5%) in 2013 up from 12.3 million (25.8%) in 1990. With an increase like this, don't you think it's time for a cure?

1.  **"Cardiomyopathy** – diseases of cardiac muscle
2.  **Hypertensive heart disease**– diseases of the heart secondary to high blood pressure or hypertension
3.  **Heart failure**
4.  **Pulmonary heart disease**– a failure at the right side of the heart with respiratory system involvement
5.  **Cardiac dysrhythmias**– abnormalities of heart rhythm
6.  **Inflammatory heart disease**
7.  **Endocarditis**– inflammation of the inner layer of the heart, the endocardium. The structures most commonly involved are the heart valves.
8.  **Inflammatory cardiomegaly**
9.  **Myocarditis**– inflammation of the myocardium, the muscular part of the heart.
10. **Valvular heart disease**

11. **Congenital heart disease**– heart structure malformations existing at birth
12. **Rheumatic heart disease**– heart muscles and valves damage due to rheumatic fever caused by *Streptococcus pyogenes* a group A streptococcal infection"

**How many of the causes above involve inflammation?**

**What is primarily responsible for inflammation?**

"There are several risk factors for heart diseases: age, gender, tobacco use, physical inactivity, excessive alcohol consumption, unhealthy diet, obesity, family history of cardiovascular disease, raised blood pressure (hypertension), raised blood sugar (diabetes mellitus), raised blood cholesterol (hyperlipidemia), psychosocial factors, poverty and low educational status, and air pollution. While the individual contribution of each risk factor varies between different communities or ethnic groups the overall contribution of these risk factors is very consistent. Some of these risk factors, such as age, gender or family history, are immutable; however, many important cardiovascular risk factors are modifiable by lifestyle change, social change, drug treatment and prevention of hypertension, hyperlipidemia, and diabetes."

To take a closer look at each one, you need to examine the risk factor I consider the most important, lifestyle. When I talk about lifestyle, I'm talking mostly about eating habits and the foods that we ingest the most, simple carbohydrates. As mentioned before, and it's something that you all know, you are what you eat. You know that sugar kills. Carbohydrates are sugars amplified. The term carbohydrate is defined as a multiple sugars and this is what makes it so dangerous. It's its ability to be turned into glucose, with little to no other nutritional value. That is precisely what makes it so deadly.

Just looking through the various causes of the different types of cardiovascular disease, was enlightening, to say the least. What I found to be a prevalent factor, throughout many of the causes for many of the diseases, was evidence of carbohydrate consumption, so I attempt to point out the fact that if this one factor was taken out of the equation of heart disease, that would change the end result of the equation.

**Only by looking at each one individually and learning, will we know;**

- **"Cardiomyopathy**– literally "heart muscle disease") is the measurable deterioration for any reason of the ability of the myocardium (the heart muscle) to contract, usually leading to heart failure. Common symptoms include dyspnea (breathlessness) and peripheral edema (swelling of the legs). Those with cardiomyopathy are often at risk of dangerous forms of irregular heart rate and sudden cardiac death. "Although the term "cardiomyopathy" could theoretically apply to almost any disease affecting the heart, it is usually reserved for "severe myocardial disease leading to heart failure." Cardiomyopathy and Myocarditis resulted in 443,000 deaths in 2013, up from 294,000 in 1990. Of all the types shown on Wikipedia, only the last one was obesity related, as "Obesity-associated Cardiomyopathy". I think doctors should consider how much junk has to be pushed with the blood, when looking at why the heart muscle weakens, not to mention the dirty blood feeding the heart muscle, weakening it from the inside as well. It's a double whammy of Macrophage/inflammation that carbs bring with them, everywhere they go.
- **Hypertensive heart disease**– diseases of the heart secondary to high blood pressure or hypertension, influence more heart disease than any other one cause. Hypertension or high blood pressure affects at least 4 billion people worldwide. Hypertensive heart disease is only one of several diseases attributable to high blood pressure. Other diseases caused by high blood pressure include ischemic heart disease, stroke, peripheral arterial disease, aneurysms and kidney disease. Hypertension increases the risk of heart failure by two or three-fold and probably accounts for about 25% of all cases of heart failure. In addition, hypertension precedes heart failure in 90% of cases, and the majority of heart failure in the elderly may be attributable to hypertension. Hypertensive heart disease was estimated to be responsible for 1.0 million deaths worldwide in 2004 (or approximately 1.7% of all deaths globally), and was ranked 13th in the leading global causes of death for all ages. Drug treatment may be needed to control the hypertension and reduce the risk of cardiovascular disease, manage the heart failure, or

control cardiac arrhythmias. High blood pressure results in 13% of CVD deaths, while tobacco results in 9%, diabetes 6%, lack of exercise 6% and obesity 5%. The very best way to avoid these conditions is to avoid that, which is responsible for high blood pressure, high starch carbohydrates like bread. Article 7 gave you an idea of how to avoid hypertension. My abstinence from carbs for the last two years has given me, for the first time in my adult life, as close to perfect blood pressure as I've ever had, 120/60. And I attribute it to the lack of carbs in my diet and my conversion to a ketogenic diet. My doctor told me I still have high blood pressure (it used to always run high). I just control it better now. Even she is astounded by what my diet has done for my health. I know what causes high blood pressure more than anything else, carbs.

- **Heart failure** often referred to as congestive heart failure (CHF), occurs when the heart is unable to pump sufficiently to maintain blood flow to meet the body's needs. Chronic heart failure (CHF) is often referred to as congestive cardiac failure (CCF) and the signs and symptoms commonly include shortness of breath, excessive tiredness, and leg swelling. The shortness of breath is usually worse with exercise or while lying down, and may wake the person at night. A limited ability to exercise is a common feature. Coronary artery disease, stroke, and peripheral artery disease involve atherosclerosis. (Remember the AGEs?) This is primarily influenced by high blood pressure, smoking, diabetes, obesity, high blood cholesterol, poor diet, and excessive alcohol consumption, which are all influenced by nothing other than carbohydrate digestion.

90% of all cardiovascular disease is preventable. Decreasing risk factors for atherosclerosis goes far to preventing most CVDs as does avoiding hypertension and of course diabetes.

"Common causes of heart failure include coronary artery disease including a previous myocardial infarction (heart attack), high blood pressure, Atrial fibrillation, Valvular heart disease, excess alcohol use, infection, and Cardiomyopathy of what many experts consider an unknown cause, I consider, ECC. These cause heart failure by changing either the structure or the functioning of the heart. There are two main types of heart failure: heart failure due to left ventricular dysfunction and heart failure with normal ejection fraction depending on if the ability of the left ventricle to contract is affected, or the heart's ability to relax is affected. The severity of disease is usually graded by the degree of problems with exercise. Heart failure is not the same as myocardial infarction (in which part of the heart muscle dies) or cardiac arrest (in which blood flow stops altogether)."

A majority of inflammation and plaque that builds up in the blood is directly due to oxidative stress and the byproducts it produces, free radicals in the form of cytokines that form macrophages, that wreak real havoc in all systems. With all the cytokine activity going on in the blood, I wonder if the influence of glucose on our hormones (hormones are what influences thyroid disease), doesn't also have an influence in thyroid disease? We know that carbs influence our hormones. We learn that in *The Payoff Of Life Without Carbs,* as well as *Carbs, Why The Addiction Is So Hard To Break,* and I touched on it in *Carbs, How They Cause AGEs.* I don't think too many studies were done on the influence that carbohydrates have on the hormones that effect thyroid disease. Other forms of heart disease display the influence of carbs a lot more, with inflammation.

- **Inflammatory heart disease**
- **Endocarditis**– inflammation of the inner layer of the heart, the endocardium. The structures most commonly involved are the heart valves.
- **Inflammatory cardiomegaly**
- **Myocarditis**– inflammation of the myocardium, the muscular part of the heart.
- **Rheumatic heart disease**– heart muscles and valves damage due to rheumatic fever caused Rheumatic fever is a disease of inflammation.

I can see where glucose plays a major part in more than a few of these causative factors. We know that glucose is the major player in high blood pressure because of the way it's digested into fat. We know that wheat has a propensity to cause muscle tics and spasms. The question I ask myself is, why can't wheat affect the heart muscle as what happens with Atrial Fibrillation when the heart starts to race for no apparent reason?

"Heart failure may also occur in situations of "high output," (termed "high output cardiac failure") where the ventricular systolic function is normal but the heart cannot deal with an important augmentation of blood volume. This can occur in overload situation (blood or serum infusions), kidney diseases, chronic severe anemia, Beriberi (vitamin $B_1$/thiamine deficiency), Thyrotoxicosis, Paget's disease, arteriovenous fistulae, or arteriovenous malformations." Viral infections of the heart can lead to inflammation of the muscular layer of the heart and subsequently contribute to the development of heart failure. Additionally, infiltrative disorders such as amyloidosis and connective tissue diseases such as systemic lupus erythematosus have similar consequences. Obstructive sleep apnea (a condition of sleep wherein disordered breathing overlaps with obesity, hypertension, and/or diabetes) is regarded as an independent cause of heart failure", when actually the direct cause of all this is the same, **ECC**.

Inflammation is a major influence in most of the various types of heart disease as well as cancer. The number one cause of inflammation is **ECC**; with the closer to obese your body is, the more inflammation you get to deal with.. We know that carbohydrates are the direct cause of body fat. We know that the most dangerous of these fats, is visceral fat, the kind your body deposits, from eating carbohydrates. Since we know all of the above, why haven't we figured out that keeping this food out of our diet will eliminate 90% of the reasons for inflammation?

I remember learning about amyloids and amyloidosis when researching cancer. It's the folding of misshaped proteins caused by glycation of cholesterol, which in turn, is caused by consumption of carbohydrates. It seems everywhere I look I see evidence of excessive carbohydrate consumption involved in the equation of too many types of cardiovascular disease. How much closer would the reduction of carbohydrate consumption bring us to controlling these epidemics? That begs the question, in who's interest is it, that we continue going down this path, we're on. What corporate industries would rather we stay on this path? Food and Drug? Where does that leave our FDA? Indebted? Or empowered? I think it's the former.

How many more have to die before people will heed these words? I know why the general public can't. I know why they don't want to pay attention to this. It's called addiction. It's called denial of addiction. The first people to deny this are quite often the ones who have it worst and are in complete denial that this would ever happen to them. This is a denial that we as a society need to face. I know. I was there. I denied it. Read my story in *About Me, How hard it is for me to appear normal..*

I weighed 205 lbs just 3 years ago. My blood pressure averaged 140/90. I controlled it with diuretics which depleted my body of potassium and calcium, both crucial micronutrients for a healthy heart. I quit bread, alone. Then I quit all wheat products. That started a cascade of miraculous things that began to happen to my health. And they all happened in beneficial ways removing any side effects (from wheat consumption), that existed prior to my conversion. I'm as normal of a person as you can get. If this can happen to me, it will happen to anyone who does the same thing that I did.

### I ask myself, why is this food still advertised as "healthy"?

This truly begs the question, if this food staple was replaced in our food supply, with something more nutritious and less glycemic, would we see a decline in the occurrences of these horrendous diseases? This is my biggest 'what if' question, what if society saw the truth in what is really going on when you eat bread and other glucose raising foods, and started to reduce their consumption of these foods, would we see a decline in these diseases? I don't just think so, I know from experience, that it will. Science says, yes it definitively will. Will addiction allow us? That's the question.

The question is, will this (food) industry allow us to do that? I seriously doubt they'll do anything about it, if it's going to hurt their business in any way. Alternatives need to be found for this food staple, not only in our diet, but in our food industry as a whole. We must make it evident, to the food industrial complex that we need to reduce our consumption of these high starch foods, if we're to remain healthy as a society. Where are the warnings: contains glucose? Where does the responsibility lie with the food industry, the grain industry in particular, those who provide the crop seed for our farmers who grow this food for us.

# Article 9

# CARBS AND ARTHRITIS

**Carbs cause arthritis?**

**Uh.....Yep!**

**You Bet!!**

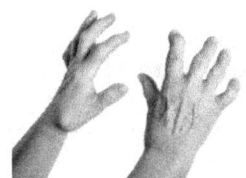
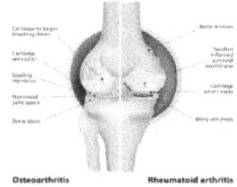

**Nothing else in the body creates inflammation, more than carbohydrates in our diet and arthritis is a disease of inflammation.**

Carbs are the foundation of inflammation. They are the sole internal source of inflammation. Inflammation wouldn't even exist (except for external injuries) without carbohydrates.

Inflammation is caused by glucose and proteins or lipids in the form of cholesterol coming together without that important signaling enzyme (hormone or cytokine) to tell them what to do and glycating. It happens because of the massive amounts of glucose in the blood. Fat, by itself, doesn't cause inflammation. It needs glucose to do that. Protein, by itself, doesn't cause inflammation. It needs glucose to do so, also.

That makes glucose, the evil villain in this drama, the drama of inflammation in the body and how it's made. Every manifestation has an equation, or a set amount of variables that make up that which is being manifested.

With that said, we're going to look at the variables that make up the equation of arthritis, the variables that cause inflammation in the body, because after all, arthritis is a disease of inflammation.

Arthritis is the expression of inflammation in the body and it shows up mostly in the joints, first, where movement takes place. That's because this is where the macrophages get deposited, where the blood flows through the cartilage where the abrasion from movement takes place.

There's another expression of inflammation in the body and it's called a common cold. The funny thing about inflammation is that because it exists everywhere the blood flows, it affects every system in the body. A common cold, for example, expresses itself with inflammation in the sinuses. I know that this may be hard to believe, but if you remove the instigator of inflammation, carbohydrates, a common cold becomes much easier to endure. Actually, common colds are not experienced in people on a ketogenic diet nearly as much as they are in carbolics, those on a carbohydrate diet. This is because of the amount of inflammation that carbs cause. Viruses may play a part in the spread of a common cold, but without the glucose in the system, the expression of inflammation can't take place. In this manner, colds and allergies are much easier to put up with, reducing the need for medication to reduce the inflammation. Unfortunately for those addicted, this can only be proven by eliminating carbs from the diet completely (which will be their fortune in the long run).

It's basically the same with arthritis, because blood flows throughout the entire body and the inflammation exists in the blood, The inflammation is going to affect every system that blood flows through, including the joints of all limbs.

**Before we can continue with arthritis, we need to know what Wikipedia says about it;**

"Arthritis (from Greek arthro-, joint + -itis, inflammation; plural: arthritides) is a form of joint disorder that involves inflammation in one or more joints. There are over 100 different forms of arthritis. The most common form of arthritis is osteoarthritis (degenerative joint disease), a result of trauma to the joint, infection of the joint, or age. Other arthritis forms are rheumatoid arthritis, psoriatic arthritis, and related autoimmune diseases. Septic arthritis is caused by joint infection."

If the definition of arthritis is joint inflammation, we know where inflammation comes from, it comes from carbohydrates, as explained in article 3 about AGEs. That makes glucose the bad actor here, because without the free glucose roaming through your blood, inflammation wouldn't exist.

It's glucose that glycates the unused proteins and fats, by attaching themselves to these cells. The glucose is looking for insulin to turn itself into fat so it can join one of the LDL particles in your blood. If it finds a protein particle or cholesterol particle (almost always LDL particles) to attach itself to, it'll do so, and this is where the problem of inflammation begins. When this happens, the glucose, glycates the cholesterol or protein and its these misshaped proteins and glycated cholesterol that forms plaque and creates inflammation.

This is where I think it gets really interesting, if the lipid that makes up the particle comes from carbohydrates, it attaches itself to an apolipoprotein B and forms LDL cholesterol to be used as fuel for the body.

If the lipid comes from fat, it associates with apolipoprotein A, the foundation of high density particles or HDL cholesterol. Learn how the HDL and LDL work in your body by reading *The value of balancing your cholesterol* and *The foundations of LDL cholesterol, apolipoprotein B*, coming up in the next articles.

It's the LDL particles that cause most of the damage because of their loose form. Hence the name, low density lipoprotein. When these particles become glycated, they are at the base of over half of all cancers, CVDs, brain damage and arthritis.

Arthritis is predominantly a disease of the elderly, but children can also be affected by the disease. More than 70% of individuals in North America affected by arthritis are over the age of 65.

This tells me that arthritis is going to happen to everyone on a carbohydrate diet, regardless of how many carbs they consume each day. Remember that 90% of the population is gluten sensitive. This is something that can only be reversed by the industry that feeds us. As long as we have to eat the food they provide us and encourage us to eat, this problem will not subside. It's in the science, the science of inflammation. This is my lasting expression of my past carbolism and it's going to be with me for the rest of my life, for there is no getting rid of it, especially considering all the carbs I fed it when I was addicted. That explains why our addiction to these vile substances must come to an end. As a society, we need to change this pattern.

The problem of arthritis goes deeper than just inflammation, though. It rides on the amount of vitamin D in the system, as well. Vitamin D is crucial to the transport of cholesterol into the cells, so it can be used.

Again, according to Pubmed; *"Vitamin D refers to a group of fat-soluble secosteroids responsible for enhancing intestinal absorption of calcium, iron, magnesium, phosphate, and zinc. In humans, the most important compounds in this group are vitamin D₃ (also known as cholecalciferol) and vitamin D₂(ergocalciferol)."*

Vitamin D deficiency is more common in people with rheumatoid arthritis than in the general population. Some trials have found a decreased risk for RA with vitamin D supplementation while others have not.

If Rheumatoid arthritis sufferers have a deficiency of vitamin D in their bodies, that tells me that vitamin D helps to control the expression of Rheumatoid arthritis by allowing the cholesterol particle admittance into the cell so it can be used. (No conductor, no admittance.)

This action prevents the cholesterol from being used and instead, becoming glycated and turned into inflammation, because with lower levels of vitamin D in the body, the arthritis is more prevalent. That tells me why lower levels of vitamin D increases Rheumatoid Arthritis. It's the one-two punch that hits everyone with arthritis; carbs raise LDL particles, raising total cholesterol throwing up flags that cholesterol must be lowered. When that's the worst thing you can do. Your cholesterol doesn't need to be lowered (that leads to disease), it needs to be balanced, so you can continue to use your cholesterol to feed your cells the nutrients they need to function properly. We'll see in article 8, The *Value of Balancing Your Cholesterol*, where you can learn how to balance yours.

"Most vitamin D is produced in our skin by ultraviolet rays acting on cholesterol; *Vitamin D₃ is produced photochemically from 7-dehydrocholesterol in the skin of most vertebrate animals, including humans. The precursor of vitamin D₃, 7-dehydrocholesterol is produced in relatively large quantities. 7-Dehydrocholesterol reacts with UVB light at wavelengths between 270 and 300 nm, with peak synthesis occurring between 295 and 297 nm.* This is what makes sunlight so important, and why vitamin D levels go down in the winter when sunlight is at its lowest with the days being shorter." That was according to PubMed.

With vitamin D actually being a fat, in the body, as it comes from cholesterol and cholesterol is made up of lipids, that makes me wonder if it comes from digested fats (carbs) or ingested fats and oils. A look at 7-dehydrocholesterol revealed nothing as to where it comes from, so I have to be content just knowing it's a lipid. Being a lipid gives it access to the cellular structure of all organs, including the skin, bones, and most importantly, your brain.

This places the importance of vitamin D even higher than what I thought before. Vitamin D is a fat that delivers calcium to your bones, making it that important to bone growth and structure. Yet it's also important in your brain, as well the rest of your body where it acts as a conductor for cell signaling proteins, cytokines and adipokines and hormones.

Again according to Pubmed; "Vitamin D receptor in the brain; It should be noted that vitamin D signaling is conducted through the VDR, which shares its structural characteristics with the broader nuclear steroid receptor family. In 1992, Sutherland et provided the first evidence that the VDR is expressed in the human brain. Using radio labeled complementary deoxyribonucleic acid (DNA) probes, the authors showed that VDR messenger ribonucleic acid is expressed in the postmortem brains of patients with AD or Huntington's disease. In a landmark study, Furthermore, the VDR is also expressed in the prefrontal cortex, cingulate gyrus, basal forebrain, caudate/putamen, thalamus, substantia nigra, lateral geniculate nuclei, hypothalamus, and cerebellum. Importantly, VDR gene polymorphisms are associated with cognitive decline, AD, Parkinson's disease, and multiple sclerosis."

Showing how important vitamin D is in the brain, it's become evident that it's as important, as the cell signaling can't take place efficiently without it, as it's the conductor. Without enough vitamin D in your system, the conduction is going to be poor, at best. Could it be that this is where cell degradation begins, and inflammation introduces its ugly face? Whether or not it is, we know that vitamin D is crucial for hormones and cell signaling proteins to get their signals through the cell membrane, as that's what conductors do, they transmit signals.

That tells me, if the pathway is blocked, due to vitamin D deficiency, the cells can't perform their intended function, because their fuel, lipoproteins can't get through the cells, due to the lack of a conductor, vitamin D, so they're left floating around in the blood waiting to be used.

This is where the problem begins because there's also massive amounts of glucose floating in the blood, waiting to be turned into fat, This gives us the equation that nobody wants, Glucose + cholesterol = glycation. Glycation is the start of inflammation.

According to PubMed; "Vitamin D lipid-lowering effects appear limited to statin-treated patients and are likely due to decreased cholesterol absorption." Cholesterol plays a much bigger part in this play, than what seemed apparent a few minutes ago. If statin drugs lower total cholesterol and vitamin D, I can only imagine what damage that is wreaking on the bodies of those who are condemned to use them. That tells me that those on statin drugs, are condemned to more inflammation, more disease, and more arthritis, can this be true? Why would the pharmaceutical companies impose that on everyone prescribed these drugs? Is it that they want more of their business?

This is exactly why it's so important to balance your cholesterol instead of just lowering it. *The value of balancing cholesterol* tells us that raising HDL cholesterol will help lower LDL cholesterol to help keep it balanced to control the inflammation by limiting the source of the inflammation, LDL cholesterol. Knowing that raising vitamin D levels can help lower LDL particles help makes it easier to lower LDL particles. Fewer LDL particles in the blood lowers inflammation lessening the effects of arthritis in the body.

Now that we know that , We also know that lowering carb intake lowers LDL cholesterol as it's carbs that create LDL cholesterol. So curbing carbs, even though it can't restore, immediately, the damage that's already been done, it can reverse its current effects, and in the future work to restore at least some of the damage. But it can only restore that which isn't already too much damaged. This again forces me to ask, why is this food even on our grocery shelves without a warning?

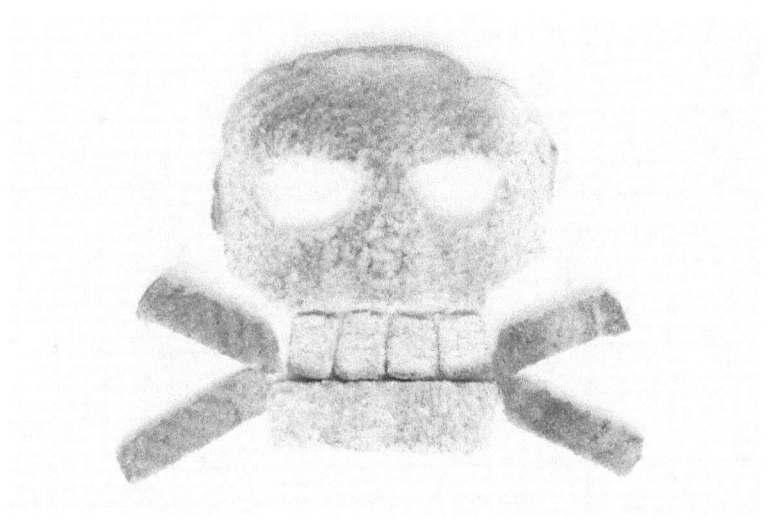

ARE YOU THINKING IT'S TIME YET?

TO CURE YOURSELF

BY CURBING YOUR CARBS

TO  BALANCE YOUR CHOLESTEROL,

AND REDUCE YOUR INFLAMMATION,

**IT'S YOUR CHOICE**

THE CURE IS YOUR'S TO HAVE

AND IT'S FREE!

## Article 10

## The Value of Balancing Your Cholesterol.

Too often I hear the phrase I've got to get my cholesterol down. People saying this think that high cholesterol is something to fear. High cholesterol isn't nearly as big of a problem as unbalanced cholesterol.

**Cholesterol is a very important part of bodily functions and plays a major impact in your health.**

**TO LOWER ONES CHOLESTEROL IS TO ENDANGER ONE'S LIFE.**

"Low cholesterol has been connected to depression, anxiety, bipolar disorder and statistically higher frequency of violent behavior, suicide, Parkinson's disease, and cancer mortality. Susceptibilities to tuberculosis and gastrointestinal infections are also associated with lower cholesterol levels. Most significantly, the death rate is doubled in older adults with lower total cholesterol and stroke and cataracts rates are higher." That was according to The Great Plains Laboratory , but you can find the same message from multiple sources, proclaiming the dangers of low cholesterol.

Cholesterol is how your body transports fuel, (lipids) to cells to fuel them. LDL particles are what fuels your cells and how you make these LDL particles is going to dictate how this fuel powers your body. If the fuel is dirty, it's going to gum up your systems. On the other hand, if it's clean, you get high octane performance out of it., with a body that heals itself.

Dr Mercola says; "The Risks of Low Cholesterol, Impaired memory and dementia are just the tip of the iceberg when it comes to low cholesterol's impact on your brain. Having too little of this beneficial compound also:

- Increases your risk of depression
- Can cause you to commit suicide
- May lead to violent behavior and aggression
  - Increase your risk of cancer and Parkinson's disease"

Whether you trust Dr Mercola or not, what he has to say about low cholesterol it true, according to the science of how cholesterol works in your body.

Unfortunately, in the United States lowering cholesterol levels has become so common that nearly everyone reading this either knows someone struggling to do so, or has struggled to do so themselves. This dangerous practice can only lead to a greater need for pharmaceuticals in the future. Stick with me and I'll show you just what I mean... .

## CHOLESTEROL IS NOT THE ENEMY

Cholesterol is essential for all animal life, each cell synthesizes it through a complex process ending with a 19 step conversion of lanosterol to cholesterol. Increased dietary intake of industrial trans fats, but not ruminant saturated fats (including cholesterol), is associated with an increased risk in all-cause mortality, cardiovascular diseases and type 2 diabetes.

"Most ingested cholesterol is esterified, and esterified cholesterol is poorly absorbed. The body also compensates for any absorption of additional cholesterol by reducing cholesterol synthesis. Biosynthesis of cholesterol is directly regulated by the cholesterol levels present, though the homeostatic mechanisms involved are only partly understood. A higher intake from food leads to a net decrease in endogenous production, whereas lower intake from food has the opposite effect." Simply stated, the more cholesterol you eat, the less you make. But because most ingested cholesterol is esterified, and ready to use, it's a much healthier fuel for the body to use. Not having sticky sugar(glucose) in it, makes it even that much healthier.

In addition to its importance within cells, cholesterol also serves as a precursor for the biosynthesis of steroid hormones, bile acids, and vitamin D. Cholesterol is crucial in the manufacture of hormones for the body's function. As vitamin D is crucial for brain function, cholesterol is crucial in the manufacture of vitamin D. This is why statin drugs that are made for lowering cholesterol, are so dangerous.

Cholesterol is your body's fuel transport system with the lipids they transport, being your body's fuel. With a substance as vital as this, why do people want to lower it? Maybe we should look at how the lipids are transported to your cells and what role that plays in the cholesterol equation.

### Cholesterol is transported inside lipoproteins

Cholesterol comes in many forms of lipoproteins, HDL (High Density Lipoproteins), LDL (Low Density Lipoproteins), and VLDL (Very Low Density Lipoproteins) just to name a few. This is where it gets a little confusing because these particles, LDL and HDL are often referred to LDL cholesterol and HDL cholesterol, when it's the cholesterol that makes up the particles. The difference is in how the cholesterol is packed in these particles. That, in turn, dictates how easy they are to glycate and start wreaking havoc in your body. I'll explain that after we learn the differences in these particles and it has to do with the building blocks of HDL and LDL particles, apolipoproteins, which we go over in article 10 *Apolipoprotein B The Foundation Of LDL Cholesterol*.

Low-density lipoprotein (LDL) is one of the five major groups of lipoproteins. These groups, from least to most dense, are: chylomicrons, intermediate-density lipoprotein (IDL), very low-density lipoprotein (VLDL), low-density lipoprotein and high-density lipoprotein (HDL), all of them, particles far smaller than human cells. In nutrition, LDL is sometimes referred to as the "bad cholesterol".

Lipoproteins transfer fats around the body in the extracellular fluid and allow fats to be taken up by the cells of the body. Lipoproteins are complex particles composed of multiple proteins which transport all fat molecules (lipids) around the body within the water outside cells. They are typically composed of 80-100 proteins/particle (organized by a single apolipoprotein B, C, E or H for chylomicrons, IDL, VLDL, LDL, the larger particles). The fats carried include Cholesterol, phospholipids, and triglycerides; amounts of each vary considerably.

LDL particles vary in size and density, and studies have shown that a pattern that has more small dense LDL particles, called *Pattern B*, equates to a higher risk factor for coronary heart disease (CHD) than does a pattern with more of the larger and less-dense LDL particles (*Pattern A*).

LDL particles pose a risk for cardiovascular disease when they invade the endothelium and become oxidized, since the oxidized forms are more easily retained by the proteoglycans. Glycation regulates the oxidation of LDL particles, chiefly stimulated by presence of necrotic cell debris and free radicals in the endothelium. Increasing concentrations of LDL particles are strongly associated with increasing rates of accumulation of atherosclerosis within the walls of arteries over time, eventually resulting in sudden plaque ruptures and triggering clots within the artery opening, or a narrowing or closing of the opening, i.e. cardiovascular disease, stroke, and other vascular disease complications.

It's easy to see now, the importance of lowering LDL. What I wonder; if lowering LDL is as important is everyone seems to think? I think not. I think it's more important to clean up the LDL in our blood, so it can work more efficiently. This, in turn, would make it a cleaner burning fuel for our bodies to use, since it's LDL particles that feed our cells. The trick here is to feed your body clean fuel, the fuel from fats, not dirty fuel, that of carbs, where the glucose makes the fat. This, in my opinion, is the basis of 80% of all of the disorders and diseases that we live with today. Especially when it comes to diseases of inflammation.

Here's the key; because it's LDL particles that feed the cells, it's vital to make sure that what they are feeding the cells is clean fuel. LDL particles that come from carbs is not clean fuel. It's dirty fuel at best. I contend that it's this dirty fuel that's creating 80% of illness and disease that I mentioned earlier.

According to The AMORIS prospective study done in March 2006 concerning stroke mortality and apoB/apoA-1 cholesterol ratios; "These observations link the apoB/apoA-I ratio to the risk of fatal stroke in a similar fashion as for myocardial infarction and other ischaemic events. Our findings indicate that the apoB/apoA-I ratio, which indicates the 'cholesterol balance', is a robust and specific marker of virtually all ischaemic events."

Low-density lipoprotein (LDL) cholesterol concentration has been the prime index of cardiovascular disease risk and the main target for therapy. However, several lipoprotein ratios or "atherogenic indices" have been defined in an attempt to optimize the predictive capacity of the lipid profile. Total/high-density lipoprotein (HDL) cholesterol and LDL/HDL cholesterol ratios are risk indicators with greater predictive value than independent levels, particularly LDL. Lipoprotein ratios have a much greater predictive power than those which include LDL cholesterol levels only.

With the advantages of HDL as opposed to the disadvantages of LDL, it's become important to know the difference in HDL and LDL because a balance in the ratio seems to be more important than anything else.

Other studies showed the same results, "LDL/HDL x 5 was a more sensitive index predicting re-infarction than total cholesterol, LDL or HDL." That to me, says what's important to know, is how to create HDL and not, how not to create LDL but how can we create clean LDL rather than the dirty ones you get from carbohydrate consumption. This will go much further than any medicine to lower total cholesterol.

HDL particles remove fats and cholesterol from cells, including from within the artery walls, (atheroma) and transport it back to the liver for excretion or re-utilization. This is what makes HDL particles the "good cholesterol", their ability to scrub your cells to remove contaminants.

Increasing concentrations of HDL particles are strongly associated with decreasing accumulation of atherosclerosis within the walls of arteries. This is important because atherosclerosis eventually results in sudden plaque ruptures, cardiovascular disease, stroke and other vascular diseases. This is why HDL particles are referred to as "good cholesterol" because of their ability to transport fat molecules out of artery walls, reduce macrophage accumulation, and thus help prevent or even regress atherosclerosis.

High LDL with low HDL level is an additional risk factor for cardiovascular disease. In a large sample of middle aged adults, low HDL cholesterol was associated with poor memory and decreasing levels over a five-year follow-up period were associated with decline in memory. It appears that low HDL leads to brain loss because of your body's inability to clean out the cholesterol from the cells, as that's what HDL's primary function is.

With all that said, it's easy to see that not all cholesterol is equal. Some is good and some is bad. Thus is the "good cholesterol, bad cholesterol mantra", which more than anything boasts the value of balancing your cholesterol, rather than lowering it. The paragraph above about HDL cholesterol says it all, increasing HDL cholesterol is a good thing, as it's "associated with decreasing accumulation of atherosclerosis within the cell walls of the arteries". As you can see, HDL, the good cholesterol is something you want in your body, according to Wikipedia who goes on to say about HDL;

The paragraph above about HDL cholesterol says it all, increasing HDL cholesterol is a good thing, as it's "associated with decreasing accumulation of atherosclerosis within the cell walls of the arteries". As you can see, HDL, the good cholesterol is something you want in your body, HDL is the smallest of the lipoprotein particles. It is the densest because it contains the highest proportion of protein to lipids. Its most abundant apolipoproteins are apo A-I and apo A-II. (A rare genetic variant, ApoA-1 Milano, has been documented to be far more effective in both protecting against and regressing arterial disease; atherosclerosis). For example, HDL and its protein and lipid constituents help to inhibit oxidation, inflammation, activation of the endothelium, coagulation, and platelet aggregation. All these properties may contribute to the ability of HDL to protect from atherosclerosis, and it is not yet known which are the most important.

The liver synthesizes these lipoproteins as complexes of apolipoproteins and phospholipid, which resemble cholesterol-free flattened spherical lipoprotein particles; the complexes are capable of picking up cholesterol, carried internally, from cells by interaction with the ATP-binding cassette transporter A1. A plasma enzyme called lecithin-cholesterol acyltransferase (LCAT) converts the free cholesterol into cholesteryl ester, a more hydrophobic form of cholesterol, which is then sequestered into the core of the lipoprotein particle, eventually causing the newly synthesized HDL to assume a spherical shape. HDL particles will increase in size as they circulate through the bloodstream and incorporate more cholesterol and phospholipid molecules from cells and other lipoproteins.

HDL transports cholesterol mostly to the liver or steroidogenic organs such as adrenals, ovary, and testes by both direct and indirect pathways. In humans, probably the most relevant pathway is the indirect one, which is mediated by cholesteryl ester transfer protein (CETP). This protein exchanges triglycerides of VLDL against cholesteryl esters of HDL. As the result, VLDLs are processed to LDL, which are removed from the circulation by the LDL receptor pathway. The triglycerides are not stable in HDL, but are degraded by hepatic lipase so that, finally, small HDL particles are left, which restart the uptake of cholesterol from cells.

The cholesterol delivered to the liver is excreted into the bile and, then the intestine either directly or indirectly after conversion into bile acids. Delivery of HDL cholesterol to adrenals, ovaries, and testes is important for the synthesis of steroid hormones.

This is where is gets interesting again; if the LDL particles are clean it's not bad cholesterol. If it's dirty, it's bad. So the LDL, "bad cholesterol" is something to either keep levels low in your body, or keep what LDL particles that you do have, clean. This is why it's important to get all your cholesterol from sources you eat, as they give you cleaner cholesterol. Cholesterol is something you don't want to make on your own, with glucose. (Remember, glucose is sticky and sticks to anything including cholesterol). When your body has to make the cholesterol, it always has the by-products of glucose in it because what it was made from, glucose and insulin.

Cholesterol that you eat comes already esterified. It's esterified cholesterol meaning, it's already been converted into an ester, ready to find an apolipoprotein C to combine with to form an LDL particle. But this particle is clean because it comes from fat, not glucose, that icky, sticky, gooey, gluey stuff. Sticky in, sticky out. Sticky glucose makes sticky lipids that make sticky cholesterol, not clean healthy cholesterol. Can you see the future need, for more pharmaceuticals, by putting dirty fuel in your body?

High density lipoproteins transfer fats from cells, and this is what makes them so important. They clean out what the LDL particles deposit into the cells. If the LDL particle is a dirty particle made up of lipids made from glucose, it's going to be a much more damaging fuel, for the cell to use. Now I can see why those on a high fat diet have so much more energy. It's the high octane fuel we use, from fats, that gives us our energy. There's nothing sticky in it to slow us down.

In your blood and the blood of all other carboholics, all of the loose floating lipids, (triglycerides, VLDL, LDL and IDL cholesterol) are more open, for glycation by loose glucose in the system, than the lipids contained in the tighter more compact HDL packets. This makes them more likely to become glycated and turned into plaque.

With that said, balancing your cholesterol seems to be much more important than just lowering your cholesterol. You really don't want to lower your good cholesterol, the HDL because of all the good it does, yet lowering the LDL with all the damage that it does, (if it's an LDL particle made from carbs), would be wise. But even lowering LDL particles is presenting a danger also, as it's the particle of fuel yet to be used. In this case, the importance lies in where this fuel comes from, carbs or fat. Carbs make dirty cholesterol. Fat gives you clean esterified cholesterol. Yet still, balance is the critical marker.

There are several ways to balance cholesterol. Certain changes in diet and exercise may have a positive impact on raising HDL levels:

- Decreased intake of simple carbohydrates
- Aerobic exercise
- Weight loss
- Magnesium supplements raise HDL-C
- Addition of soluble fiber to diet (Curb the starchy carbs and trade them for fruits and vegetables)

- Consumption of omega-3 fatty acids such as fish oil or flax oil
- Increased intake of saturated fats
- Consumption of medium-chain triglycerides (MCTs) such as caproic acid, caprylic acid, capric acid, and lauric acid.
- Removal of trans fats from the diet

Most saturated fats increase HDL cholesterol to varying degrees and also rai
Most saturated fats increase HDL cholesterol to varying degrees and also raise total and LDL cholesterol. A high-fat, adequate-protein, low-carbohydrate ketogenic diet may have similar response to taking niacin (vitamin B3) as described below, lowered LDL and increased HDL through beta-hydroxybutyrate coupling the Niacin receptor 1.

According to the BMJ; "Saturated fats are not associated with all cause mortality, CVD, CHD, ischemic stroke, or type 2 diabetes, but the evidence is heterogeneous with methodological limitations. Trans fats are associated with all cause mortality, total CHD, and CHD mortality, probably because of higher levels of intake of industrial trans fats than ruminant trans fats".

The best saturated fats you can eat are Medium Chain Triglycerides (MCTs). MCTs from coconut oil as well as milk fats increase HDL cholesterol. MCTs passively diffuse from the GI tract to the portal system without requirement for modification like long-chain fatty acids or very-long-chain fatty acids(longer fatty acids are absorbed into the lymphatic system). In addition, MCTs do not require bile salts for digestion. Patients who have malnutrition, malabsorption or particular fatty-acid metabolism disorders are treated with MCTs because MCTs do not require energy for absorption, use, or storage.

Based on 5 separate studies; MCTs can help in the process of excess calorie burning, thus weight loss. MCTs are also seen as promoting fat oxidation and reduced food intake. Other studies show increases of HDL particles when MCTs are added to the diet. According to BMJ (British Medical Journal)

Medium Chain Triglycerides come from Coconut oil, Palm Kernel oil and all dairy fats. That means that butter and cheese can actually help you lose weight and balance your cholesterol. How great is that? You can go back to eating butter with healthier consequences than eating margarine.

Coconut milk is rich in medium-chain fatty acids (MCFAs), which the body processes differently from other saturated fats. If MCFAs are used in a diet to replace long-chain fatty acids (LCFAs) such as animal fats they may help promote weight maintenance without raising cholesterol level." "Coconut milk contains a large proportion of lauric acid, a saturated fat that raises blood cholesterol levels by increasing the amount of high-density lipoprotein cholesterol" Like coconut milk, coconut oil is high in *Lauric acid*.

Medium-chain triglycerides are generally considered a good biologically inert source of energy that the human body finds reasonably easy to metabolize. They have potentially beneficial attributes in protein metabolism, but may be contraindicated in some situations due to a reported tendency to induce ketogenesis and metabolic acidosis. However, there is other authority reporting no risk of ketoacidosis or ketonemia with MCTs at levels associated with normal consumption. Due to their ability to be absorbed rapidly by the body, medium-chain triglycerides have found use in the treatment of a variety of malabsorption ailments. MCT supplementation with a low-fat diet has been described as the cornerstone of treatment for Waldmann disease. MCTs are an ingredient in some specialized parenteral nutritional emulsions in some countries (not USA). Studies have also shown promising results for neurodegenerative disorders (e.g. Alzheimer's and Parkinson's diseases) and epilepsy through the use of ketogenic dieting.

MCFA (chain lengths of 10 carbons or less are found in greatest concentrations in coconut oil, approximately 14% by weight but can also be found in butter ( approximately 9.2%) and palm kernel oil (approximately 7.2%) MCT oil has been taunted as a potential weight-lowering agent.

According to the US National Library of Science, The "Weight-loss diet that includes consumption of medium-chain triacylglycerol oil leads to a greater rate of weight and fat mass loss than does olive oil."

Thirty-one subjects completed the study (body mass index: 29.8 ± 0.4, in kg/m²). MCT oil consumption resulted in lower endpoint body weight than did olive oil. There was a trend toward greater loss of fat mass and trunk fat mass with MCT consumption than with olive oil. Endpoint trunk fat mass, total fat mass, and intra-abdominal adipose tissue were all lower with MCT consumption than with olive oil consumption.

So the question here, is not how do we lower cholesterol, rather, it's how do we make clean LDL particles that won't contaminate the cell structure, like the dirty LDL particles do? The best way to do that it to make the LDL particles out of cleaner sources than glucose, the foundation of body fat. Using body fat for LDL particles is what's responsible for all the disorders associated with apoB. That's because this fat's foundation is glucose, a sticky, gooey, gluey, substance that makes the fat it turns into almost as sticky, gooey and gluey is its foundation. This is not clean cholesterol and it gums up the cells, arterial walls and everything else it has a relationship with. It's not hard to understand how this cholesterol can be responsible for so many disorders. Dirty fuel has a tendency to ruin the engines that burn them.

All that I've researched shows that it comes from glucose. The glucose from starchy carbohydrates. As I explained in *Carbs! The Newly Discovered Death Sentence* and *Diabetes Control*. It all has to do with the digestion of carbs. These fats are apportioned to the visceral fat around the belly instead of glycogen you can use for immediate fuel. and this is where it's formed into LDL with the help of Ribosomes from your liver. This is also where it becomes so dangerous, but you'll have to read about it in my next article. Lowering the blood lipid concentration of triglycerides helps lower the concentration of small LDL particles, because fatty-acid rich VLDL particles convert in the bloodstream into large loose LDL particles.

In my attempt to find what fats cause LDL, I've found nothing to suggest that eating fat causes the formation of LDL. But, on the other hand, I've found plenty of data that suggests where this kind of fat comes from. That's in my next article, about Apolipoprotein B.

It makes sense then, if you want to stop the production of LDL, you need to stop the production of triglycerides, the fuel that feeds it, and the best way is to stop that, is to curb the high starchy carbohydrates from the worst offenders, grain based foods. The guiltiest of the group is wheat, followed closely by corn, then rice and oats. All grain based foods are at the top of this list, along with starchy vegetables like potatoes, parsnips and carrots, although carrots do have some nutritional value, like beta-carotene. All the others just don't carry enough nutrition to counterbalance the load of starchy carbs you get, with them.

If you're not ready to give up your carbs, there are alternatives, to help you lower you LDL, Niacin ($B_3$), lowers LDL by selectively inhibiting hepatic diacylglycerol acyltransferase 2, reducing triglyceride synthesis and VLDL secretion through a receptor HM74 and HM74A or GPR109A. " A ketogenic diet may have similar response to taking niacin (lowered LDL and increased HDL) through beta-hydroxybutyrate, a ketone body, coupling the niacin receptor (HM74A).

Statin drugs are made to lower LDL also, but I can only recommend to steer clear of those, as they cause too many problems in their action of lowering LDL. As a certified caregiver, I've seen, too often, the ravages this drug commits the body to. They are nothing short of devastating. In every case of a patient I took care of, the patient died prematurely from the side effects of these drugs. It seems to me that in our attempt to cure ourselves, we're killing ourselves. Cholesterol is just too important to lower.

So, a MCT ketogenic diet can not only help you balance your cholesterol but it can help you lose weight and keep it off forever. Who knew that coconut oil or coconut milk could be so healthy? Who knew that butter could be so healthy? I certainly didn't. but I do now.


Because ketogenic diets are made for calorie restriction and this next point deals with calorie restriction, I can see the benefits here, as well, for added BDNF for brain growth, increased Nrf2 for anti-oxidant production. If you don't know about the brain growth or anti-oxidant boost of calorie restriction, we'll be going over that in *The benefits of life without carbs*. I'm just beginning to understand the benefits of the MCT ketogenic diet and how much healthier it's kept me. And if it can keep me that healthy, it can keep all those who venture to try it just as healthy. We're all running around on high octane fuel, because of the lack of carbs in our diet and this is why I put my faith in fat.

## Don't you think it's time for a cure?

I offer this one to you freely!

*Spices That Heal*

Found at the link on the website, there are a multitude of spices that can help with a range of problems that carbohydrate digestion cause like high cholesterol and high blood pressure, spices like Bay Leaf can help balance your cholesterol, as described on *Spices That Heal, "Research on humans showed that after one month, the bay leaf group had up to 26 % reductions in blood sugar! They also showed approximately 35 to 40% reductions in LDL cholesterol and a jump in the good HDL particles by about 25%!"* Hibiscus flower is excellent for controlling high blood pressure and makes an excellent tea. Just looking halfway through the list, I came across another half dozen spices that can all help balance cholesterol. What an excellent resource.

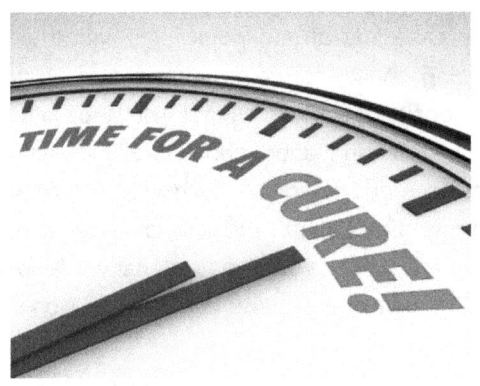

**I just love free Cures.**

# Article 11

# THE FOUNDATION OF LDL PARTICLES, APOLIPOPROTEIN B

When it comes to LDL particles, what I have discovered tells me to be aware of Apolipoprotein B. But before we can look at Apolipoprotein B we need to know what these apolipoproteins are.

Apolipoproteins are proteins that bind lipids (oil-soluble substances such as fat and cholesterol) to form lipoproteins. They transport the lipids through the lymphatic and circulatory systems. Apolipoproteins are the foundation of all cholesterol particles.

This is the start of cholesterol, these dictate how cholesterol is carried in your blood stream. They're the foundation for HDL particles as well as LDL particles and they also dictate how the cholesterol is going to perform in your body. It gets interesting because it's what kind of cholesterol they're going to make that dictates how they are classified, high density low density, very low density, intermediate density or chylomicrons.

There are six different kinds of apolipoproteins with the two major types of apolipoproteins being Apolipoproteins A and Apolipoproteins B, with the latter forming low-density particles. Most of the other apolipoproteins form high-density lipoprotein ("good cholesterol") particles. These proteins consist of alpha-helices and associate with lipid droplets reversibly. During binding to the lipid particles these proteins change their three-dimensional structure. There are also intermediate-density lipoproteins formed by Apolipoprotein E. These find VLDL and LDL particles to join.

The lipid components of lipoproteins are insoluble in water. However, because of their detergent-like (amphipathic) properties, apolipoproteins and other amphipathic molecules (such as phospholipids) can surround the lipids, creating the lipoprotein particle that is itself water-soluble, and can thus be carried through the blood.

These amphipathic or amphiphilic properties tell me why we lose weight when we exercise. This is how the body disposes of used fats, with HDL particles. It's the LDL particles that feed the fats into the cells and it appears that this is where the problem with Apolipoprotein B comes into play, Apolipoprotein B is sometimes a dirty or glycated protein, meaning that it's bent, so that it can't be used properly. This is when glucose attacks the lipid before it can be encapsulated into cholesterol.

There are six classes of apolipoproteins and several sub-classes. Most all are HDL building apolipoproteins except for Apolipoproteins B and E. Those are the ones that builds LDL and IDL respectively and they're the ones that are the genesis for so many ailments and diseases. This tells me that most apolipoproteins are made in the intestine, however the Apolipoprotein B is formed in the liver. I have to wonder if this is where its problems begin. Is this why Apolipoprotein B is the basis for so many diseases? Knowing that it's LDL particles tells me that they're more easily invaded by glucose and that is what glycates the cholesterol, which is where most of the problems with disease begin.

- A (apo A-I, apo A-II, apo A-IV, and apo A-V) - High density
- B (apo B48 and apo B100) – Low Density
- C(apo C-I, apo C-II, apo C-III, and apo C-IV) - High density

- D - High density
- E - Low density
- H - High density

Exchangeable apolipoproteins (apo A, apo C and apo E) have the same genomic structure and are members of a multi-gene family that probably evolved from a common ancestral gene.

Hundreds of genetic polymorphisms of the apolipoproteins have been described, and many of them alter their structure and function. In particular, apoA1 is the major protein component of high-density lipoproteins; apoA4 is thought to act primarily in intestinal lipid absorption. That tells me that Apolipoprotein A is manufactured in the intestine. Apolipoprotein synthesis in the intestine is regulated principally by the fat content of the diet.

Apolipoprotein B is formed in the liver, the organ that filters the blood; Apolipoprotein synthesis in the liver is controlled by a host of factors, including dietary composition, hormones (insulin, glucagon, thyroxin, estrogens, androgens), alcohol intake, and various drugs (statins, niacin, and fibric acids). Apo B is an integral apoprotein whereas the others are peripheral apoproteins.

It appears that the foundation of HDL type cholesterol particles or Apolipoproteins A, C, D, E, and H comes from the fat you eat, whereas the foundation of LDL type of particles (Apolipoprotein B), comes from many sources, as it's made in the liver. Maybe it's polluted Ribosomes that make the protein cells, since they're made in the liver, than in the intestine, like the Apolipoprotein A. Because the liver cleans all the toxins out of the blood, maybe some of the toxins get deposited in some of the Ribosomes the liver manufactures for protein synthesis. I don't know if this is the start of "bad cholesterol" or not, but that's not the point. The point is that there are too many variables in the manufacture of Apolipoprotein B, from dietary choices to alcohol consumption to hormones and drugs that you take, to make it a steady source of reliable apolipoproteins for consistently healthy cholesterol, thus, "Bad Cholesterol". This is why, when it comes to LDL, what I have discovered tells me to be aware of Apolipoprotein B and what creates it. *So, what does create* Apolipoprotein B?

The biggest factor in regulating Apolipoprotein B, is dietary choices, including alcohol consumption. This would entail consumption of all sugars, since we know that fats are responsible for Apolipoprotein A,C,E and H. There are only three basic food groups, fats, proteins and carbohydrates, we know that fats are good because they create Apolipoprotein A, proteins are good because they are the basic building blocks or our bodies, leaving sugars or carbohydrates to create Apolipoprotein B, the basis of most diseases.

## That tells me to Stay Away From All Sugars.

Dietary choices and Alcohol consumption both have to deal with sugar in the diet, because the fats in your diet go to make the foundation of HDL particles. It's the sugar in the diet, or the carbs in the diet that make up the Ribosomes that make the proteins that are the foundation of LDL particles. Put plainly, carbs in the diet create LDL particles, fat in the diet creates HDL particles. That explains why this dirty LDL is so dangerous, its base proteins are apolipoproteins made in an organ that filters blood for the body as well as being formed by particles made from dirty lipids, those which come from glucose.

Apo lipoprotein B  is a protein that in humans is encoded by the *APOB* gene. "Apo lipoprotein B is the primary  apolipoprotein  of chylomicrons, VLDL, IDL, and LDL particles, which is responsible for carrying fat molecules (lipids), including cholesterol, around the body (within the water outside cells) to all cells within all tissues. It is the primary organizing protein of the entire complex shell enclosing and carrying fat molecules within the cholesterol particle. It's the base component of the particles and is absolutely required for the formation of these particles. What is also clear is that the ApoB on the LDL particle acts as a ligand for LDL receptors in various cells throughout the body.

Through mechanisms only partially understood, high levels of ApoB, associated with the higher LDL particle concentrations, are the primary driver of plaques that  cause vascular  disease (atherosclerosis),  first  becoming symptomatic as heart disease, stroke & many other complications following decades of progression. There is considerable evidence that concentrations of  ApoB  and  especially  the NMR  assay  (specific  for  LDL-particle concentrations) are superior indicators of vascular/heart disease's causative factors than either total cholesterol or LDL-cholesterol (as promoted by the NIH in the 1970s). However, cholesterol, and estimated LDL-cholesterol by calculation, remains the most commonly promoted lipid test for the risk factor of atherosclerosis. ApoB is routinely measured using immunoassays such as ELISA or nephelometry. High levels of ApoB are related to heart disease.

It is well established that ApoB100 levels are associated with coronary heart disease, and are even a better predictor of it than is LDL level. A naive way of explaining this observation is to use the idea that ApoB100 reflects lipoprotein particle number, independent of their cholesterol content. In this way, one can infer that the number of ApoB100-containing lipoprotein particles is a determinant of atherosclerosis and heart disease.

ApoB100 is found in lipoproteins originating from the liver (VLDL, IDL, LDL). Importantly, there is one ApoB100 molecule per hepatic-derived lipoprotein. Hence, using that fact, one can quantify the number of lipoprotein particles by noting the total ApoB100 concentration in the circulation. Since there is one and only one ApoB100 per particle, the number of particles is reflected by the ApoB100 concentration. The same technique can be applied to individual lipoprotein classes (e.g. LDL) and thereby enable one to count them as well.

This tells me that it's not the amount of cholesterol in your body that's important. It's the number of ApoB100 lipoproteins floating around, that's important. So, what do I need to look out for to keep from building this ApoB100, in my system? What causes ApoB?

"Apolipoproteins are of great physiological importance and are associated with different diseases such as dyslipidemia, cardiovascular and neurodegenerative diseases. Apolipoproteins have therefore emerged as key risk markers and important research targets yet the function of apolipoproteins has not been fully elucidated." That's according to Mabtech, they go on to say, "Apolipoproteins are proteins that bind hydrophobic lipids in the blood and help solubilize them. Together with phospholipids, apolipoproteins form lipoprotein particles into which different lipids can be packed. Apolipoproteins have pivotal functions as structural components in lipoprotein particles, ligands to receptors and co-factors to enzymes. Lipoprotein particles are necessary for transportation of lipids used for energy supply and for synthesis of hormones, vitamins and bile acids. ApoB and apoE are important in the transport of dietary and endogenous lipids to peripheral tissues for energy supply, whereas apoA1 is crucial for the returning of excess cholesterol from peripheral tissues back to the liver. Apolipoproteins such as apo E and apo J are also important for the transportation of lipids in the brain."

With all the different kinds of cholesterol, just lowering it seems to me, to be a little counterproductive. Cholesterol is your body's fuel. It's what each cell burns.

I can see where high levels of HDL particles in the blood to clean out the cholesterol in the cells is more important than high levels of LDL particles to feed the cells, as it's important to keep the flow of cholesterol through the cell, in order to keep cholesterol from building up in the blood and getting glycated by any loose glucose in the blood looking for insulin to enter a cell.

Balancing cholesterol in this respect  is much more important than just lowering cholesterol, whether it be LDL particles or HDL particles. In my opinion, lowering cholesterol, whether it's LDL or HDL,  is like signing your death warrant. The only cholesterol that needs to be limited in the body is that cholesterol that's made of the lipids that glucose and insulin make.

- Apolipoprotein A - the genesis of HDL healthy cholesterol, comes from fats in the diet
- Apolipoprotein B - the foundation of LDL bad cholesterol, comes primarily from carbs in the diet

All cholesterol is so important for fat transportation in our bodies as well as hormone balance, vitamin D production and removing fats from the body, my question is, why would anyone in their right mind, want to lower it when a good balance of cholesterol is so much more important.

## IT'S TIME:

TO CURB YOUR CARBS

TO  REDUCE YOUR BAD CHOLESTEROL

TO REDUCE YOUR PLAQUE

AND INFLAMMATION.

# Article 12

# GASTRIC BYPASS AND THE LOSS OF GHRELIN

When I heard from a dear friend that he wanted to go through gastric bypass surgery, because he couldn't get his weight under control, my heart sank. I thought he's heading into a life time of more illness and disease, just because he can't control his carb intake. One wouldn't think that losing part of their stomach could hurt that much, when in all actuality, you're looking at cutting one of your most important lifelines. That is, if you don't want to be addicted to pharmaceuticals for the rest of your life. I'm beginning to wonder why this procedure would ever be recommended,

I wouldn't be so concerned about this, if one of the effects of this surgery didn't involve loss of one of your most influential hormones, Ghrelin. Post surgical data show a reduction in the amount of Ghrelin in the stomach of bypass surgery recipients. This one factor alone could severely limit your ability to fight off future illnesses and disease.

Your stomach doesn't just hold food to be digested, it produces one of the most important hormones for your health, Ghrelin. If you take away the source of this hormone, you're taking away future health.

I touch on this in *The Payoff of Life Without Carbs*, and it has to do with control of your hormones. If you let your hormones control you, you're going to be subject to leptin's influence and your hormones are going to follow their own path of least resistance. This is going to continue, to force you to feed them, more carbs.

However, if you'd rather control your own hormones, you'll learn the value of Ghrelin resistance. This will allow the Ghrelin to build up in your system where it can perform its magic, the magic of building a bigger brain and boosting anti-oxidants.

Ghrelin is first and foremost a growth hormone, as well as a hunger hormone, but it also serves many other functions. These functions include but are certainly not limited to, the following attributes;

- Ghrelin promotes intestinal cell proliferation and inhibits apoptosis during inflammatory states of oxidative stress. It also suppresses pro-inflammatory mechanisms and augments anti-inflammatory mechanisms, thus creating a possibility of therapeutic use in various gastrointestinal inflammatory conditions, including colitis, and sepsis. Animal models of colitis, ischemia reperfusion, and sepsis-related gut dysfunction have been shown to benefit from therapeutic doses of Ghrelin. It has also been shown to have regenerative capacity and is beneficial in mucosal injury to the stomach.
- The hippocampus plays a significant role in *neurotrophy*: the cognitive adaptation to changing environments and the process of learning and it is a potent stimulator of growth hormone. Animal models indicate that Ghrelin may enter the hippocampus from the bloodstream, altering nerve-cell connections, and so altering learning and memory. It is suggested that learning may be best during the day and when the stomach is empty, since Ghrelin levels are higher at these times. A similar effect on human memory performance is possible.

Although the vast majority of neurons in the mammalian brain are formed prenatally, yet parts of the adult brain (for example, the hippocampus) retain the ability to grow new neurons from neural stem cells, a process known as neurogenesis. Neurotrophins are chemicals (family of proteins) that help to stimulate and control neurogenesis. BDNF being the most important of these.

Looking at the attributes above, Ghrelin not only supports anti-inflammatory mechanisms, but it's this last attribute that sets it apart from all the other benefits that this diet provides, as it promotes neurotrophins in the brain which in turn is the start of new neurons. In other words it makes the brain grow. That means that going hungry turns on factors in your brain that actually make it grow. BDNF is just one of these neurotrophins that I talk about in *MY Life Without Carbs* article.

So Ghrelin not only tells you when to eat, it also inhibits cell death, it helps control pain and disease by controlling anti-inflammatory mechanisms as well as encouraging our brain to grow through a process of neurogenesis, the growth of new brain cells.

It's this last factor that intrigues me the most. This means that I can grow new brain cells, something that I thought was lost 30 years ago after my severe closed head injury. I used to think that brain cells couldn't grow back, when in all actuality, they're growing all the time, through neurogenesis, (at least for those who want them to grow).

Ghrelin is the hormone of choice when it comes to controlling inflammation. Reducing the amount of it in the body will do little more than increase any expression of inflammation and that includes arthritis and pain, the worst expression of inflammation. Why would anyone want to increase their pain?

Ghrelin is such an important hormone in the body, I can't understand why anyone would want less of it in their body. It protects the body from so much it'd be a downright shame to lose anything that supplies it. I can't think of a trade off that would make that worth it.

## How to increase Ghrelin

This may indicate the healthiest benefit of being on a ketogenic diet, the ability to resist the influence of Ghrelin on your urges to eat.

Building Ghrelin in your body is not the easiest thing to do. It requires effort. There are several way to build your Ghrelin, some easier than others, but all effective.

For me the easiest way was to exercise, but exercise wasn't getting me to my other goals. It was increasing my brain power, but it wasn't helping me to lose weight. It wasn't until I decided to give up carbs myself that I finally reached my weight goals and this turned out to be the healthiest manner in which I can increase my brain power. This, to me, is evidence of the biggest difference of a carb diet and a keto diet.

It was when I went on the keto diet, my brain growth seemed to multiply because it was 23 months after my switch that I published the site that led to this book. When you compare that to the length of time it took me to write my post about myself, the difference is astounding. I attribute that to a lack of carbs in my body to muck things up.

**The differences between a high carb diet and a low carb (keto) diet.**

A carbohydrate diet, through the glucose it uses to make fat, provides the following damages and benefits for your body;

**Damage**

- increases glucose in the body
- which creates fat
- which creates plaque,
- inflammation,
- high blood pressure
- arthritis
- heart disease
- cancer
- Alzheimer's
- Parkinson's
- dementia
- lack of hormonal/emotional control
- more expression of leptin in the body
- more pain
- more hunger
- less overall energy

**Benefit**

- Tastes good

- Satiates quickly
- Quick temporary energy

In comparison, a ketogenic diet provides for the body;

## Downside

- No quickly satiating food to eat

## Benefit

I lay out most of these benefits in *My life without carbs*;

- Limited glucose in the system to glycate or muck things up
- More energy
- Longer lasting energy
- Larger expression of Ghrelin's benefits in the body

    1. Bigger brain through brain growth (extra BDNF in the brain)
    2. Anti-oxidant growth (extra Nrf2 to amp up anti-oxidants)

- Weight maintenance is natural
- Low to no body fat
- Less plaque in the blood
- No heart disease
- No cancer
- No arthritis
- Less inflammation
- Less pain
- Less expression of a common cold
- Fewer mosquito bites

I used to get mosquito bites all the time. It seemed that mosquitoes flocked to me just to get some of my blood. Now. I rarely get bitten. When I do get a mosquito bite, a seldom notice it, as it doesn't itch as much as it used to. That is evidence to me, of a lack of willingness of my body to get inflamed, from a mosquito bite. How sweet it is.

Becoming Ghrelin resistant is in my opinion, the biggest benefit of being on a ketogenic diet. This allows Ghrelin to work more of its magic in my body.

When one balances the benefits versus the damage each diet inflicts on the body, it's not hard to see the benefit of the keto diet over the carb diet.

## When I hear of gastric bypass surgery now, I think, Where is the sense in this?

It's amazing to think about what some people will unknowingly force themselves to endure, just for the vague perception of an easy path out of their dilemma, when all they have to do, is curb their carbs.

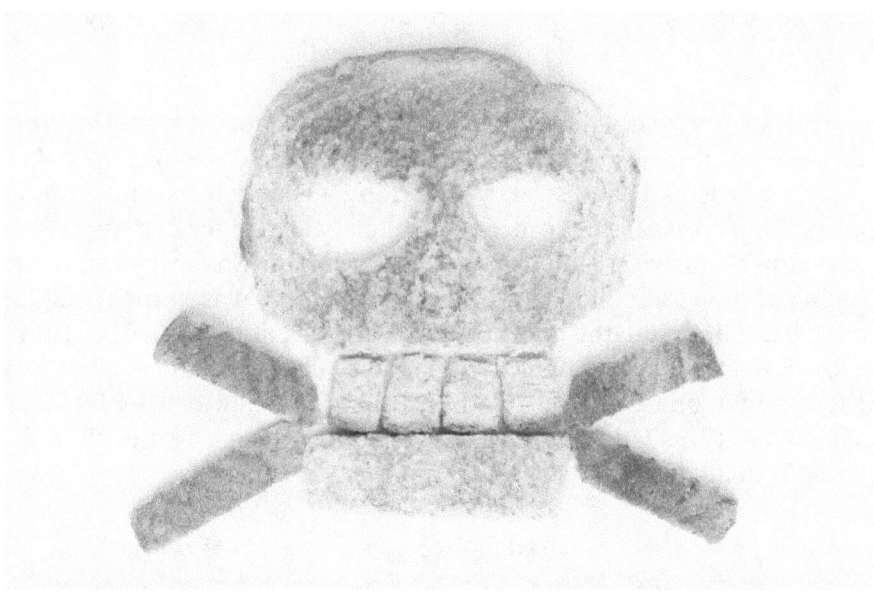

# ARTICLE 13
# WHY NO OUTRAGE, WHY NO WARNINGS

When stupid people do stupid things, it has a tendency to catch people's attention. As with the recent acts of terrorism. Stupid people acting as bullies, being stupid. Their tactics only work when we agree to be as stupid as them, and be afraid. That's how bullies work, through fear, and if you don't fear them, their tactics won't work.

We're all outraged about terrorism and the number of lives it's taken and continues to take, which is understandable. Acts of terrorism are almost always emotionally senseless acts of violence done simply for political or personal gain. There's absolutely no rationality to it, except for greed.

Why is it, we're so afraid of terrorism? Terrorism in itself might be responsible for almost 0.3% of all deaths. We stand a much more chance of suffering and dying just by getting on the freeway, or easier yet, by simply continuing to eat our comfort foods.

According to Wikipedia "as of 2002, the percentage of deaths, from intentional injuries, i.e. war, violence and suicide was 2.84%". Terrorism as bad as it is, has yet to claim as many lives each year, as either heart disease or cancer or obesity or type 2 diabetes or Alzheimer's disease, alone! As bad as terrorism was last year, it still hadn't claimed a million lives. yet cancer alone, was responsible for over 8.2 million deaths or 14.6% of all human deaths in 2012. That's 22,465 deaths per day, worldwide, due to cancer. Heart disease was the number one cause of death with 17.3 million deaths in 2013. That was 47,397 deaths per day. In 2002 it was responsible for 29.34% of all deaths." In 2013, it was up to 31.5 %.

1/2 of all cancers can be linked to excessive carbohydrate consumption. 1/2 of all cardiovascular diseases can be linked to excessive carbohydrates consumption.

**ECC - Excessive Carbohydrate Consumption is responsible for as much as 42% of all deaths, a minimum of 24 million deaths each year.**

I know that sounds outrageous. I think it is outrageous. Yet, I never hear any outrage, about the number of people's lives that these diseases claim. Allow me to show you exactly how these grain based foods - breads, cereals and pastas (high starch carbs), if removed from the diet, would reduce the occurrence of these diseases by a minimum of 80%. Yes, a reduction of 80% in the occurrences of these diseases, in aggregate, simply by removing the excessive consumption of high starch carbohydrate foods from our diet. Why isn't this treated as a medical condition? It has a very simple cure, don't eat these types of food anymore.

Reducing the occurrence of these diseases would have a couple adverse side effects to our society, reducing the need for the medical community to treat these diseases and eliminating the need for diet companies. I haven't researched how big of an industry the diet and health industry is, but it would definitely have an effect on it, and it might force a lot of people to seek alternative employment.

I tend to wonder if this is why most doctors won't discourage their patients from consuming them? I think mostly, it's just a matter of ignorance, They don't know, or they don't want to know because of their own addiction. (Once you kick the addiction, you can see its influence in those who doubt this concept, the most.) Maybe it's because of their patients addiction to it and their fear of losing their patients to their addiction. This happens when the addiction speaks louder than a patient's personal health, the patient will find a doctor who will treat them with pills or surgery instead of giving up their addiction. That in itself, is proof of the addictive nature of this food.

### 4,100,000 Preventable Deaths From Cancer Each Year!

### Where's the outrage?

When you add cancer deaths of over 8.2 million in 2012, half of which are linked to diet, to the 17,3 million deaths from heart disease, 90% of which are preventable, that adds up to 25.5 million deaths each year, 77% of which are completely preventable. That's 19.67% of all deaths, worldwide, each year are completely preventable and it doesn't count the deaths from any of the other diseases that come from being obese or from having type 2 diabetes or type 3 diabetes, Alzheimer's disease and dementia, which are completely preventable also.

After experiencing what I've experienced and researching what I've researched, I can link 1/2 of all cancers directly to diet. With that said, combine 4.1 million deaths from cancer that could be saved with the 90% of the 17.3 million deaths from heart diseases (15,570,000) and you get a total of 19,670,000 deaths each year that are completely preventable, simply by making a simple yet major diet change. Don't yield to the addiction of this food and buy into the lifetime of need to purchase drugs to combat the diseases that these foods cause.

### 5,000,000 Preventable, Undignified Deaths

### From Alzheimer's Disease Each Year!

### Where's The Outrage?

It's hard to say exactly how many people die from Alzheimer's disease. With a life expectancy of just six years after diagnosis and with between 21 million and 35 million (as of 2010), having the disease, that means that there will be approximately another 30 million deaths (give or take 3-5 million) from Alzheimer's disease alone, within the next 6 years. That's 5 million each year, 90% of those diseases are preventable. I never hear any outrage about the number of people's lives that these diseases claim.

### 15.570,000 Preventable Deaths From Cardiovascular Disease Each Year!

### Where's The Outrage?

According to Wikipedia, *"Cardiovascular diseases are the leading cause of death globally. This is true in all areas of the world except Africa. Together they resulted in 17.3 million deaths (31.5%) in 2013 up from 12.3 million (25.8%) in 1990." "It is estimated that 90% of CVD is preventable. Prevention of atherosclerosis is done by decreasing risk factors through: healthy eating, exercise, avoidance of tobacco smoke and limiting alcohol intake."* 90% of 17.3 is 15.57 which attributes to 15.57 million deaths, due to heart diseases that are preventable. That, to me is nothing short of astounding, yet where's the outrage?

Although relatively few die from obesity alone (usually because the obesity leads to something worse first), it leads into so many other diseases, that it is indirectly attributable to more deaths than many of these other diseases. Type 2 diabetes, obesity's first disease of death, is what leads into many cancers and heart diseases alone and is why its danger is unparalleled. That's why its control is paramount. If you can control type2 diabetes, you can control every disease it plays a part in. And, it plays a part in most of the deadliest diseases; half dozen cancers, half dozen cardiovascular or heart diseases. And most importantly, it happens in the ones that kill the most people.

Looking at just cancer and cardiovascular disease, they're responsible for more than 25.5 million deaths a year as of 2013. Half of those deaths are due to high carbohydrate consumption, either directly of indirectly. Usually it's indirectly and that is where the trouble lies. Because it is indirectly, it's practically unseen. It was unseen until Dr Davis and Dr Perlmutter uncovered all the evidence. Studies were done and the results (evidence) were quietly stored away for years, with little notice that the studies that produced the evidence ever got published or even announced that they existed.

But there was enough evidence there to influence these doctors to write two books about the danger, *Wheat Belly* and *Grain Brain.* I had already quit eating bread before I read Wheat Belly, but as I read it, it was validating everything that was happening to my body, since I gave it up. *Wheat Belly* led me to *Grain Brain,* which gave me the tools that I needed to piece this article together.

But I must give credit where credit is due. Dr Daniel Amen had persuaded me to give up bread after reading his book *Use Your Brain to Change Your Age.* In his book, he spent more time talking about eating a healthy diet, than any other one thing. At least, that was his lengthiest chapter and he had mentioned to go easy on starchy carbohydrates. It was Thanksgiving 2013 and I weighed 195 lbs at the time, 40lbs more than what I carry now.

After working out extensively for 6 years and not being able to get past the first 30 lbs I lost, in the first month, I decided that it must be my diet. I was eating healthy, very healthy, I thought. It wasn't until I quit eating bread that I found out just how unhealthy it really was. After losing 20 lbs in one month after quitting bread, I decided to give up all grains. When I mention bread, I'm talking about all bread and cereal products, including pasta, crackers and breakfast foods. If it was made of wheat, I wouldn't touch it.

In only one month I dropped to a weight, lower than what's prescribed for my height (175 lbs), I was at 165 lbs when I decided to quit all grain foods. I lost another 10 lbs, down to 155lbs. That's about where I "hover" now. I say hover because my weight fluctuates with what I'm doing with my diet. Today, for example, my weight is down to about 151lbs, because I've been on a calorie restriction diet for the last 45 days since I started writing this blog and subsequently, into a book. This action alone has been more beneficial for my brain, in particular, than anything I've ever done for it, in my lifetime. Of course it's done wonders for my body and my immune system. When I go hungry I'm creating Ghrelin in my stomach. I can feel the hunger pangs right now, but I'd rather sit here and write, than get up and get something to eat.

I've learned that it's those hunger pangs that tells me my stomach is creating the Ghrelin that activates BDNF in my brain which in turn is building me a bigger and better brain. Everything I've done in the last 45 days has virtually proven what this diet can achieve, something a carbohydrate diet can't. When you read my about me page, and compare that to what I've accomplished in the last 45 days since I started this blog, it's astonishing. At least it is to me. I have never been able to do anything like this before in my entire life. Nobody ever thought I could ever do this after my brain injury 31 years ago. I never thought I could do it. I had always thought, brain cells don't grow back. At least it had made a nice excuse for me, for all the fubars I was responsible for.

That was until I read Dr Perlmutter's book *Grain Brain* and learned that you actually can grow brain cells. I learned that thinner people have bigger brains and that calorie restriction helps build brain cells and new neural networks to connect those cells. It just takes the right formula, a formula that doesn't include any grains or starches.

**High starch carbs just don't have enough nutrition to compensate for the overload of glucose they pour into your system.**

The system it starts with is your digestive system. Then it moves to your circulatory system where it can affect every other system, and then your brain, pancreas and kidneys and eventually most all other organs, until it give us the statistics above. Since the most ubiquitous forms of these diseases involve inflammation, and these foods are the major cause of inflammation, doesn't it make sense that if you removed these foods from the diet, you would remove a major cause of the diseases that are influenced by it?

## Why are they still promoted like they are?

## Where's the recommendation from more doctors to stop eating it?

## There's absolutely no rationality to it, except addiction.

# Where's the outrage?

# PART III

# BREAKING THE ADDICTION

# ARTICLE 14

## HOW TO CUT BACK

The best way to start cutting back on your carb intake, is to stop buying the foods that you find them in. Without any high carbohydrate food around, you're forced to find alternative foods to eat and snack on.

**The best benefit of discontinuing the consumption of carbohydrates, is the lack of a need to keep eating them.**

Once the addiction wears off and your body discovers that it can live without carbs, miraculous things begin to manifest. The longer you stay off the carbs, the more miraculous these manifestations become, until you begin to experience life as it is supposed to be experienced, illness and disease free and full of energy.

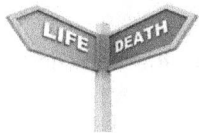

*It's your choice!*

But to just stop buying carbs, isn't stopping the consumption, because if you're like me, you have to use up what you have in your pantry. You can't just throw it all out, you have to use it up, so you don't waste it. That's addiction speaking, which we'll get into in *Breaking The Addiction*. But when it comes down to curbing your carbs, not having them around is a priority. You don't leave alcohol lying around reformed alcoholic's home, unless they've broken the addiction. For the same reason, you can't leave any carbs lying around the house waiting to be eaten, if you haven't broken your addiction. That can take years. It all depends on how hard the bug bit you.

For true addicts, there's two theories on this;

- If you can afford to throw out what breads you have in your pantry, you'd be far better off, than if you didn't. Consumption of what you have left, means that you'll only be adding to the inflammation, it causes. Continuation of this consumption will also bring on any multitude of illnesses or disease that you would NEVER experience if you didn't ingest this food to begin with.

- If you can't afford to throw it out, and have to eat it, because of financial hardship, you have two courses to consider, either damage your health by continuing to eat it, or save your health and give your carbs to the dog. If you must keep damaging your health , by continuing to eat it, slow down your consumption of it, to slow the intake of the sugars that are so deadly. This way, they won't affect your blood glucose as much, and this is what is so dangerous about eating carbs. It's the roller coaster ride that these carbs put our blood glucose through. You eat carbs, your blood glucose rises. After a couple hours, your blood glucose falls again, making you hungry again and ready to pack in more carbs, simply to raise that blood glucose. Hence, the carbohydrate roller coaster ride. Everyone on a carbohydrate diet, all ride this ride, for there is no waiting line for it. It's ready for us to take any time we want to. It's no wonder that this is causing our obesity epidemic that the whole world is experiencing today. (This is also manifestations of the genetic modifying of wheat, and other grains.)

For those of us who've kicked the addiction, there's only one clear choice, and that to throw everything out.

Unfortunately, this doesn't tell us what we should be replacing those lost calories with, so I'll make a couple of suggestions as to what you can do, to fill your stomach, then I'll give you a list of what you can't eat, if you want your body to experience these benefits;

- Eat high fiber carbs like fruits and vegetables. I list fruits here, because of the problem of satisfying our sweet tooth. In order to cut back on all the sugars that we ingest, it's easier to do, if we keep the simplest of these carbs (fructose) in our diet, for a while, at least until we wean ourselves off of the killer sugar, glucose. Fructose can be just as deadly, but because of its nature of being a 1 molecule sugar, it's digested by the liver and not on a cellular level. This means that it doesn't need insulin to be digested, and therefore doesn't affect the pancreas as much as a diet high in glucose will. Fructose just ruins the liver. A look at any wino will tell you that.

- Transition from carbs to more protein and fats in your diet. To cut the carbs, you need to replace those lost calories with healthier calories, like those from fats and protein. This will do several things to your body that are very beneficial, like reducing your weight, first and foremost, which will help you from contracting diabetes. You'll experience a decrease in any chronic pain, arthritic pain or headaches that you have to deal with, as well as experience a reduced threat of cancer and cardiovascular disease, just to name a few. Your benefits may be greater or less depending on the level of addiction that you have to deal with now. I can almost tell you, just from just looking at you, at what level of addiction you're at. The worse it is, the harder it is to kick. But also, once it's kicked, the bigger the benefits will be. Knowing this, is the secret to killing carbs.
- When you feel like a snack, which will reduce over time as your body adjusts to a low carb, *Keto diet*, turn to cheese, yogurt, raw nuts, High fiber vegetables like celery and broccoli.
- Cheese is an excellent source of protein and fat. Cheese is a MCT, medium chain triglyceride, which are great for weight control. Because all milk fats are MCTs, that means, all milk fats can help you lose weight. That also makes whole milk, cream and butter healthier than low fat, 1% or skim milk. I'm sure you never thought that eating high fat dairy products could help you lose weight, but it's true, they can.
- Raw nuts are packed full of protein, essential fats (which offer more calories per gram of food, than what carbs do), and best of all, fiber to help clean out your digestive system. Raw nuts have it all, protein, healthy omega 3 fats, fiber, you can't find a much better all around food.
- Eggs eggs may be one of the best sources of nutrition. They're packed with protein, good fats and essential oils, B-complex vitamins and essential minerals. More nutrition comes in just one egg, than what you can get out of 6 loaves of bread.
- First and foremost, don't drink your calories. When you drink your calories, it's always in the form of either fruit juice, soda, soft drinks, or alcohol. All of these beverages carry with them an enormous amount of sugar. The sugars in beer make it tops for all foods on the glycemic index, making it the most dangerous of any carb source. It upsets the delicate balance of your of sugar and cholesterol levels in your body, more than any other food. It's this balance that's so important to maintain, simply because this balance is what regulates the amount of plaque that the sugar causes, when it glycates your cholesterol. This is just the beginning or your death sentence. The continuation of it takes place with every sip of beer you drink, every sandwich you eat, every bagel you eat, every crescent you eat, every pancake you eat,,,, Are you starting to get the

picture? It's OK if there are still a lot of question in your head, now. That's good. I've at least done what I set out to do, to get you to thinking about the kind of foods that you put into your body to sustain it, because this is going to take a lot more examination, to be able to come to any viable, workable solutions for getting off of these things.

Whatever you think, don't allow the phrase low carb, or Paleo, or *Keto diet* scare you. Ketogenic diets are not for unhealthy people as much as they are for healthy people. Everyone who has an intolerance (allergic reaction) to wheat, gluten, gliadin or any of the other substances found in these grains, will experience the unhealthy consequences of a carbohydrate diet, so I'm going to give you a partial list what foods contribute to a high carbohydrate diet, more so than anything else.

**Foods that are harmful;**

- **bread** and all bread products
- **pasta**
- **rice in all forms**
- **corn in all forms, sweet, pop, meal, flour, powder, chips**
- **oatmeal in all forms,** quick being the most dangerous
- **Cream of wheat**
- **any cereal**, including granola, muesli, Wheaties, etc even special K
- **chips of any nature,** whether they be corn chips, multi-grain chips, potato chips, tortilla chips, it doesn't matter.
- **crackers**
- **pastries**
- **snacks of any grain**
- **Energy/Cereal Bars**
- **Breakfast Bars**
- **frozen breakfasts**
- **frozen meals and entrees**
- **ALL processed foods**
- **potatoes**
- **parsnips**
- **Ice Cream**, unless it's sugar free (then you get to deal with the artificial sweeteners)
- **Fresh and frozen juices**, they nothing but concentrated sugars. What other nutrition juice has, isn't worth the trade-off of the amount of sugars it puts into your system.

- **frozen waffles**
- **pancakes**
- **hash browns**
- **coffee creamer – powder or liquid**
- **any sandwich with bread or bun** use lettuce in place of bread
- **Most all breakfast foods except bacon, sausage and eggs**

**Most Dangerous;**

- **cookies**
- **Pop Tarts**
- **soda pop**
- **energy drinks**
- **alcohol**
- **beer (highest on the glycemic index)**

You cannot eat these foods, and expect to stay healthy. They change your blood sugars too much. They're way too high on the glycemic index. That's why you need to transition your diet to foods higher in protein and fat. You body needs calories, so consider, what is the best source of calories?

**Carbs have 4 calories per gram, fat has 9 calories per gram.**

**Which of these foods is more efficient, is what you should be asking yourself.**

What this basically means, is that you don't need as much food to get the same amount of energy out of what you eat. This, to me, is the smoking gun that proves how much healthier a diet high in fats is, compared to a diet high in carbohydrates.

This alternative to a carb diet, is a keto diet, or ketogenic diet. With fat being more than twice as efficient as carbs, it's a wonder that we still eat them. I've been on a MCT ketogenic diet for the last two years and I can't say enough about what it's done for my health. My weight came down 60 lbs from a high of 215 lbs 8 years ago, when I started working out. I lost the first 30 pounds in the first month just from water loss. The nice thing about water loss is, that is it includes a good supply of body fat, that comes with it. Fat is water soluble in the body and when your body expels the water, fat comes with it. My problem was that I couldn't drop my weight any further, until I changed my diet, two years ago, when I gave up the wheat products and all other grain foods. When I did that, my excess weight just magically disappeared. Within 4 months, I was 15 pounds lower than my prescribed weight, feeling great with far more energy than I've ever had. This is the biggest benefit to a *Keto diet,* more energy. I've got more energy than I've ever had. I've got so much energy, I just wish I knew about this before.

Other benefits of a Keto diet can be found in a myriad of sites around the web extolling the virtues of ketogenic diets. I've given you a few links in the post on the website, I used for this article, for your research. I hope you do research everything in this article and inform me of what isn't correct. The only way you'll know for yourself how dangerous this food is, is by vetting what you read, not only here, but in every other article you read about this subject.

The more I investigate, the more I find that disturbs me, like why does the food industrial complex still advertise this food as being healthy? Why do they advertise it as being high fiber? Why is it still advertised, that whole grains are healthy, when they're not? All of this makes me wonder, just how far will this industry go, to keep poisoning us, just so they can continue to rake in their profits. This brings us to our next problem, why didn't we know about this before? Again, this is something that will have to continue, later in part three in the book.

I know how hard it is to quit eating this food, 'cause I did it. You can read about my transformation in *Weight Loss*. It was the hardest thing I ever had to do. But with some perseverance, I did it, I noticed the change after about 1 month of abstinence. It was like a weight lifted off my shoulders all of a sudden. The room seemed brighter. All my senses felt crisper and more alive. Everything came easier, standing up, walking, sitting down, even getting out of bed was easier every morning. Everything I was experiencing and beginning to experience proved to me, the value of keeping this food out of my diet. It proved it in such a way, that I'm now doing my level best to convince the rest of my family and the world, just how dangerous this grain is. My continued use of this diet, has not only made my general health better, most importantly, it's improved my brain functions to a level I never thought imaginable. By converting my brain over to ketones instead of carbohydrates, it's allowed me to actually grow my brain, and more importantly my brain functions. My thinking has actually improved quite substantially...even with my disability still affecting me. Crosswords come easier. Names are easier to remember, even though I still have massive amounts of memory loss, due to my head injury. (The real reason I started and continue this lifestyle.) Even with the severity of my disability, having to live with the loss of short term memory, that not only blocks memories, it blocks reasoning and judgment due to the damage done to my pre-frontal cortex, from the strokes that I had, 31 years ago, I've been able to overcome a major portion of what I lost. (I still get to live with the knowledge, that I'll never get back the mental ability, that I had before.)

By using fat as a source of energy, I don't have to spend nearly as calories digesting my food, because fat is so much more of an efficient fuel. By needing less food, to create the calories I need to fuel my body, I can allow my stomach to go empty for a much longer time now. I don't have to feed it every 2 hours. I often go as many as 12 or 16 hours without eating anything. 24 hour fasts, are nothing for me to complete, now, quite comfortably even. In short, keto=life carbs=death.

Converting to a state of ketosis has allowed my body to actually go hungry for extended periods of time, without loss of energy or mental faculties, (alertness, clearness of mind, etc) or experiencing emotional roller coaster rides because of the fluctuations in my blood sugar. I am not controlled by my hunger. I control it. I don't worry about any of that because I don't have the blood glucose flowing through my system, that creates that *E-ticket* ride. I do this because I can't afford to get sick. I can't afford the medications. I can't afford the hospitalizations. I can't afford the testing, the procedures, the surgeries, the doctor visits, the specialists visits, and worse yet, I can't afford to be any more disabled than I am right now. For my story your have to read this account of my disability, *'How hard it for me to appear normal'*, that I keep for my medical records. It's already part of my medical records at Cigna, in Mesa, AZ. My doctors know what I have to live with, and even they, are convinced that this "high fat" diet that I started on, close to 2 years ago, is the healthiest diet that I could be on. I have a secret technique that I use. You'll see that coming up in article 15.

# ARTICLE 15

## WHY THE ADDICTION IS SO HARD TO BREAK

The biggest piece of the puzzle, that influences our motivations to keep this addiction, keeps us also, from enjoying freedom from the ravages, of this devious destroyer of energy, emotional control, senses, health, wealth, sensibility, sanity, and ultimately life. And it is why this addiction is so hard to break? And believe me, it's a hard piece to place. I think simply because there are so many facets to this piece. That is what we're going to look at in this article. Oh Boy! This may take a while.

It starts with the way it effects our blood sugar again. Sugar satiates the body quicker than any other food because of the effect it has on our blood glucose. It's the raising of the glucose that releases a feel good neurotransmitter, **serotonin** that tells your body to relax and feel safe.

According to Wikipedia; "Serotonin (/ˌsɛrəˈtoʊnɪn/, /ˌsɪr-/) or 5-hydroxytryptamine (5-HT) is a monoamine neurotransmitter. Biochemically derived from tryptophan, serotonin is primarily found in the gastrointestinal tract (GI tract), blood platelets, and the central nervous system (CNS) of animals, including humans. It is popularly thought to be a contributor to feelings of well-being and happiness."

It's this contribution of serotonin to our feelings of well being and happiness, that make us behave either rationally, or irrationally. It's this one little factor, in my estimation, that is where many of our problems begin. Because of the outside influence on our emotions and feelings of well being and happiness, from fluctuating glucose levels in the blood, you no longer have full control over them. The drop in serotonin, is responsible for making us act differently when our glucose levels are low, rather than when our glucose are high. This is what causes more irrational behavior than anything else, other than maybe, chemicals in our environment and food supply. On second thought, it has to be the biggest contributor, because I'm still subject to pollutants in the environment and food supply, but I'm not subject to the effects of glucose in my system effecting my serotonin levels. My emotions are much more rational than what they were, when I was on a carbohydrate diet. Fluctuating serotonin in my system seldom happens because glucose is not present, to make those serotonin levels fluctuate. My MCT keto diet doesn't alter my emotions and feelings of well being, because of the lack of glucose, it allows in my diet, to put into my system. Fact is, it allows very little glucose to get into my blood because of the lack of carbohydrates, in this diet.

Because of that, my emotions don't fluctuate as much as they used to, when I was on a carbohydrate diet. This in turn, means that every thought, every action, everything I speak, is done more rationally, than if I were still on a carbohydrate diet of any sort. This would not be possible if my body weren't in a state of ketosis. (Thank you, Dr Perlmutter!) You don't have to take my word, alone, you can ask anybody whose body is in a state of ketosis. They'll tell you the same thing, That their emotional control has developed far more, than it ever did, as a carboholic.

I theorize that serotonin plays a major part not only in our emotions, but in our desires, also. It has to. If it can influence our emotions, how can it not influence our desires? It's this influence to our desires that influences our behavior. If carbs influence the amount of serotonin in our systems, wouldn't carbs then, influence our desires, and behavior? With all this outside influence in our behavior, wouldn't it make sense, that this outside influence, also plays a major role, in the behavior of everyone in the world? It has to. Doesn't it make sense, then, if you were to reduce the outside influence in our behavior, everybody would be able to think more rationally. Wouldn't more rational thinking  throughout the world lead to less violent destruction, and war, worldwide?

But that still doesn't say enough about why it's so hard to break this addiction. That's just the biggest, most important reason. We need to look at, as many reason as we can, to help, as many people as we can, break this deadly cycle of carbolism.

Carbolism is like any other addiction, only worse, because we were all sold this bill of goods that "this is wholesome, healthy food you should be eating". So, we ate it. and we ate a lot of it. We based our diet on it. We still eat it. We consume more bread products in our diet than anything else, because we were told to. We'll continue to eat it, until everyone realizes, how dangerous, this food really is. This addiction we've thought for years (even in the medical community), was really supposed to be healthy for us. The problem is, it isn't. It hasn't been healthy for us, for the last 40 years, at least. Since genetic modification has worked its way into our food supply, studies have shown major changes in our health. Studies have shown an increase in brain degenerative diseases, about the same time that genetically modified grain, slipped into our diet. Alzheimer's has grown exponentially in the last 40 years, and many scientist, are still trying to understand why. There were also, studies showing increases in diabetes and obesity, increase in cancer, increase in cardiovascular disease and digestive disorders. And, most of this was done under our noses, without us even knowing about it. Shame on us. For the last 40 or so years, this food has been unhealthy for us, but because of the influence that this food has on our serotonin levels, we've allowed ourselves to get and continue to be addicted to it.

It's this continuation of addiction, throughout our society, that makes it so hard to break, our individual addiction to it. It's the continuation of all the advertising telling us we should still be eating this pseudo food, that's driving this addiction. What drives all of the advertising, is corporate power, simply trying to make as much money as they possibly can for their stockholders.

This is where the difficulty in breaking the addiction, begins, at the corporate level. Because advertising influences our choices so much, corporate America exerts enormous amounts of control over us. With the introduction of sugar into our diet, it makes it even easier, for them to accomplish this. I wonder why the food and drug industrial complex, keeps pushing the American people to their limit in what they can withstand, every time they advertise their killing foods.

What does everyone do on Thanksgiving day? What do you do? If you're like everyone else, you sit and watch football, the biggest advertising venue in our society, is football. What do you do while you're watching the football games on TV? If you're like everyone else, you're eating chips of some sort, and drinking soda or beer. This is when your blood glucose levels are at their highest, making your serotonin levels also at their highest, influencing a major portion of your behavior. You're feeling good. You see the advertising, you may be even ingesting the same thing you're seeing the advertising for. How do you think this is going to make you feel? What do you think it going to make you believe? That these substances are good for you? That you should be ingesting them? Naturally! this is how everyone feels. it's because of that glucose in everyone's systems' influencing their thoughts, emotions and behavior. Is it any wonder that they're addicted? This is how corporate America controls our emotions, thoughts and behavior. Remove the carbs, remove the addiction. The problem here, is that you have to break the addiction, it's that crucial.

# CORPORATE AMERICA KEEPS AMERICA
# AND THE WORLD ADDICTED

Corporations realize this. They don't want you to break your addiction. They do everything in their power, to keep you addicted. They have to. It's in their best interest to keep their stockholders happy, and the only way to do that, is to be making money, and lots of it, for higher returns in the stock market. It's the nature of business. Not even knowing that they are killing their customers, is enough, to influence them into realizing that this is a downhill road that they're on. This road is so steep, that it can and will lead, ultimately, to death of our society. Archeologists in 3050 from another planet in another galaxy, will stumble across our planet and find it an empty orb that shows evidence of civilization, but no life, because of the poisons that we continue to feed ourselves.

This is why corporations need to realize that they're killing their customers and that they're making all of their customers diabetic and sick, simply to make an extra buck, because of the excess sugar in their products. They put them in because it satiates so fast. People who ingest their products, like them immediately, making them return customers for life, or, at least, until the next best thing comes along to satiate the appetite. This behavior is completely understandable on a carbohydrate diet, which is ever so prevalent, in a all parts of the world. Maybe, corporations know what they're doing. After all, most do.

Maybe, they do realize what they're doing to the public. After all who buys their medicine, to fight all the illness and disease that this food source causes? Who designs the crop seed for the farmers to grow it?

Prior to the turn of the century, in the 80s and 90s, corporations like Monsanto, the world's biggest crop seed company, owners of companies like DeKalb Genetics Corporation, Delta & Pine Land Company, and Calgene, companies that all provide crop seed for farmers to grow the food that America puts on its tables, decided to merge their business together with pharmaceutical companies. Monsanto merged with Pharmacia and Upjohn, around the turn of the century. Their company is responsible for Celebrex, the arthritis medicine. I can't help but wonder, if they already knew about the devastating effects of their food products? Did they know that their products were actually causing arthritis? Did they know they were peddling death and disease, at that time? It seems to make sense that if they would want to increase the pharmaceutical business, there's no better place than to start than where the most impact would be, at the grocery store, where their customers buy their food to feed their addictions.

One could almost make the claim that corporate America is trying its best to keep us addicted to their "cash crop", to keep us buying their pharmaceuticals. If so, this is one trap I refuse to fall into. This is one major ruse on the American public, that's killing Americans right and left. Yet There's no outrage and worse yet, no warnings.

 Anyone who's broken this addiction to the carbohydrate diet and has allowed their body to go into ketosis, knows exactly what I'm talking about. Since they've broken the addiction of the fluctuating glucose in their bodies, their serotonin doesn't fluctuate, and thus their thoughts, emotions and behavior isn't influenced as much as that of someone on a carbohydrate diet. Their thinking is much more rational. Their thinking will never be influence by their diet, simply because of the lack of carbs in it. In other words, there are not driven by their hunger, like everyone else, who's on a carb diet.

If they have other opinions, it's usually because the addiction is still talking. I understand how hard it is to break. The hormonal conversation everyone has with themselves every minute of every day is what's driving this addiction. And it's being done at the request of an industry that's simply trying to stay in business and make some money at the same time....or so they say. This is where our food industrial complex plays their part in our addiction.

They've  learned how to use these foods' most powerful form of influence known to man, hormonal influence. It's the type of influence the victim has no control over, because of the hormonal control. Hormones have a nasty way of controlling our behavior, by blocking receptors in our brain. By blocking these receptors, those hormones have complete control of its victim. In this case the victim is the American people and it's spreading throughout the whole world in its forms of obesity and diabetes. This is one trap I refuse to walk into again. I crawled out of this trap and I certainly am not going to fall back in again. I can't help but think of the WHO and their song, "We won't be fooled again". At least, I won't ! I broke the addiction.

Is this trap corporate America is selling us worth falling into? They sell us their food products, which everyone loves to eat, because their addictive.

In turn, they expect us to buy their pharmaceuticals, after their food gives us the diseases that they're responsible for.

All this illness, is what they're banking on us to buy into, so they can sell us their more pharmaceuticals.

I refuse to.

Even though I with the rest of America, including most of my family, have been sucked into this scam, I refuse to participate anymore.

It's your choice to cure yourself,

to fight the addiction

or continue playing their game

and continue buying their drugs!

I DON'T HAVE TO, MY ADDICTION IS GONE

# ARTICLE 16

# THE PAYOFF OF LIFE WITHOUT CARBS

How often have you ever felt like you just couldn't control yourself? How often have you ever felt like your emotions and decisions were under the control of someone or something else? You knew there's something wrong, but you just can't place your finger on it, you just couldn't determine exactly what it is that was wrong, but you knew something was. You're not alone. This happens to almost everybody (except for those on a low carbohydrate diet). When this happens, it more than likely is your hormones. Your hormones are the governing agents in your body. They dictate when you're hungry and when your not. They dictate how much to eat and when to stop. Being on a high carbohydrate diet turns control of your hormones over to the food you're eating instead of keeping it under your control.

This is the biggest benefit of living a life without carbs' influence on your body. It begins to manifest itself when hormones come back under your control and not that of your high carbohydrate diet. Once carbs are out of the equation, and no longer influencing your hunger hormones, that leaves the door open for you to control your own hormones and in doing so, control how these hormones work within your body. The two most important hormones, as far as hunger and your body mass are concerned, are Leptin and Ghrelin.

Leptin and Ghrelin are the two hormones that regulate your digestive system, by telling you when you're hungry and when you're not, so that's what we're going to look at in this article.

According to Nora T. Gedgaudas, an acclaimed nutritional therapist, *"Leptin essentially controls mammalian metabolism."*Leptin decides whether to make us hungry and store more fat or to burn fat. When your stomach is full, fat cells release leptin to tell your brain to stop eating. This is your body's brake for the fork to mouth syndrome. Dr

Perlmutter goes on to say in *Grain Brain* that "millions of Americans qualify as bona fide members of the leptin-resistant club. It's practically a given if you've been eating a high carb diet and don't sleep well." A few of the signs of leptin resistance; being overweight, unable to lose weight and keep it off, constantly craving comfort foods, fatigue after meals, feeling hungry all the time or at odd hours of the night, desire to snack right after a meal, problems sleeping to name a few. For the complete list, read *Grain Brain*. Leptin resistance is not a condition to strive for. Its leptin resistance that leads to overeating and it's a very common condition while on a high carbohydrate diet.

Leptin is the hormone that tells you when to stop eating. It's called the satiety hormone, but that's not what's interesting about Leptin. What's interesting about Leptin is that it's formulated in your body fat. That means, the more body fat you have the more Leptin you'll have.

According to the New England Journal of Medicine; "Serum leptin concentrations are correlated with the percentage of body fat, suggesting that most obese persons are insensitive to endogenous leptin production."

Wikipedia goes on to say, "Although leptin reduces appetite as a circulating signal, obese individuals generally exhibit a higher circulating concentration of leptin than normal weight individuals due to their higher percentage body fat. These people show resistance to leptin, similar to resistance of insulin in type 2 diabetes, with the elevated levels failing to control hunger and modulate their weight."

**It's this Leptin resistance that gives control of your hormones over to the foods that you love to eat so much, the foods that really control it, high carbohydrate wheat and grains.**

Ghrelin, on the other hand, is the hormone that signals your brain that you're hungry. According to Dr Perlmutter, Ghrelin is the yin to leptin's yang. This hormone is secreted by the stomach when it's empty and increases your appetite. As much as leptin tells you to stop eating, Ghrelin is the one that tells your, brain it's time to eat.

Ghrelin is first and foremost a growth hormone, as well as a hunger hormone, but it also serves many other functions. These functions include, but are certainly not limited to, the following attributes ;

- Ghrelin promotes intestinal cell proliferation and inhibits apoptosis during inflammatory states and oxidative stress. It also suppresses pro-inflammatory mechanisms and augments anti-inflammatory mechanisms, thus creating a possibility of its therapeutic use in various gastrointestinal inflammatory conditions, including colitis, ischemia reperfusion injury, and sepsis. Animal models of colitis, ischemia reperfusion, and sepsis-related gut dysfunction have been shown to benefit from therapeutic doses of Ghrelin. It has also been shown to have regenerative capacity and is beneficial in mucosal injury to the stomach.

- The hippocampus plays a significant role in neurotrophy: the cognitive adaptation to changing environments and the process of learning and it is a potent stimulator of growth hormone. Animal models indicate that Ghrelin may enter the hippocampus from the bloodstream, altering nerve-cell connections, and so altering learning and memory.

- It is suggested that learning may be best right before lunch, during that time of day and when the stomach is empty. since Ghrelin levels are higher at these times. A similar effect on human memory performance is possible.

- Although the vast majority of neurons in the mammalian brain are formed prenatally, parts of the adult brain (for example, the hippocampus) retain the ability to grow new neurons from neural stem cells, a process known as neurogenesis. We already know how good Neurotrophins are for you. Remember the BDNF?

Looking at the attributes above, Ghrelin not only supports anti-inflammatory mechanisms, but it's this last attribute that sets it apart from all the other benefits that this diet provides, as it promotes neurotrophins in the brain which in turn help the brain to produce new cells. In other words it makes the brain grow. That means that going hungry turns on factors in your brain that actually make it grow. BDNF is just one of these neurotrophins that I talk about on the *MY Life Without Carbs* page.

So Ghrelin not only tells when to eat, it also help control pain and disease through controlling anti-inflammatory mechanisms as well encouraging our brain to grow by encouraging neurogenesis, the growth of new brain cells. It's this one factor that intrigues me the most. This means that I can grow new brain cells, something that I thought was lost 30 years ago after my severe closed head injury. I used to think that brain cells couldn't grow back, when in all actuality, they're growing all the time, through neurogenesis, (at least for those who want them to grow).

The question, therein lies, how do we encourage this neurogenesis? I hinted to that in the previous paragraphs and Ghrelin plays an important role in it. But something else just as important influences brain growth, and that's exercise. This is what Dr Perlmutter talks about, when he mentions that our ancestors ran for their food in primitive times as well as ran for their lives. It was this action (exercise) that set us apart from other species. We could not only run hungry, we could run longer and harder because of the diet we were on, as a species, at that time (carbs weren't part of our diet at that time). But they are now. What's worse yet? They're in our diet in abundance. And what's even more, worse yet, is that we live a sedentary life style, and it's this life style coupled with an insatiable appetite for high carbohydrate foods that's causing this obesity epidemic as well as diabetes epidemic, and that of all of the other disease that go with it.

The way I see it - high carbohydrate diet + sedentary life style = obesity, small brain, disease and death. Low carb diet + exercise = longer life, bigger, smarter brain and better immunity to fight against disease.

This one attribute, in my estimation, is the most important attribute of eating a low carb diet. Dr Perlmutter puts it this way, the fatter you are the smaller your brain and what we've just looked at proves that. It also proves that the thinner you are the larger your brain is likelier to be. To me, that says, those who can't break their addiction to the carbohydrate curse, are destined to be dumber than those who can break this addiction. In writing this entire book in the last four months, this action has proven this fact to me, that it is possible to expand our brains and thereby expand the capabilities or our brains. Thank you Dr. Perlmutter for helping me to realize and understand this little secret that I use to build my brain, I love going hungry. Technically, it's called calorie restriction. Every time I start to feel hunger pangs, my mind reminds me that I'm building up Ghrelin in my system, which in turn, is building my anti-oxidants and fortifying my brain with BDNF.

We all know that exercise is good for you, but did you know before today that it helps to grow your brain cells? What you probably didn't know, was that, hunger can produce similar results in helping your brain to generate new brain cells. This to me is what's so exiting. Just by going hungry, I'm encouraging my brain to generate new brain cells, as well as well as encouraging my body to easier fight illness and disease by boosting my immune system, by boosting my anti-oxidants exponentially. WOW! How good can this be? All I have to do is to stop eating the foods that cause this kind of behavior in my body and I can be rid of the worry of most everything listed in my first post, *Carbs, The Newly Found Death Sentence That's Ages Old.*

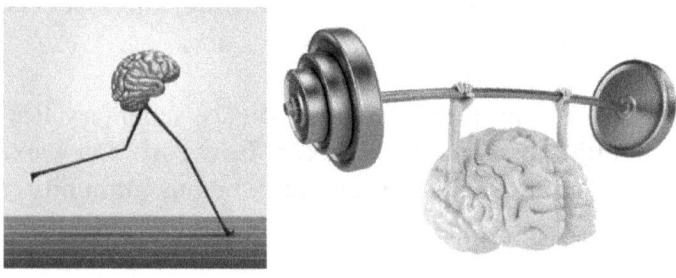

# ARTICLE 17
# MY LIFE WITHOUT CARBS

This is the best part of my journey, getting to share with you, all of my experiences, since I first gave up this horrid food. My first impulse is to think, I can't say enough about the benefits I've received and experienced from being on this ketogenic diet. But, I'm going to try to lay out as many of them as I can, explaining how it's benefited me, and more importantly, how I can save money by allowing those benefits to continue, by remaining on my keto diet. This, to me, is the most important part, of why I'm doing this.

The first benefits I received, I hinted to in my **last article**, so I'll list those *"enlightenment feelings"* that I first felt, here also. I call them *enlightenment feelings*, because of the weight they lifted off my shoulders, when I suddenly realized that I had complete control of my weight. And because I had complete control of my weight, I had much better control of my health. It actually took about a month for the *enlightenment* to come. But once it came, I knew it, and I knew it firmly. It may have been the most liberating experience I've felt since I rode my motorcycle from coast to coast, border to border, and then some. But, that was 35 years ago before my severe closed head injury changed my life.

After spending 29 years gaining weight, from a relatively sedentary life, after living with hemiplegia for 29 years from the two strokes I had in 1984, after living with chronic pain for 20 years (pain bad enough it became nauseous at times), after more than twelve years of opioid medication to fight the pain, along with antidepressants, and a multitude of other drugs and supplements meant to counteract the side effects of the opioid medication (weight gain, constipation, dull senses, growing dumber each day, prostate enlargement and too may others to list here), after countless acupuncture sessions, after more nerve blocks than I ever should have had, after searching for any drug, any device - mechanical or electrical - every therapy, and even after researching all surgical options, I'd had enough. The opioids did nothing but make me fat, lazy and stupid, and I just couldn't take it anymore. I decided 2 years ago, that I was going to stop eating bread, and that was it. I was still going to keep eating other carbs, but I wasn't going to eat bread, or anything that had any type of *"bread product"* in it. I told my family that, and I don't think they believed me. I really don't think anyone in my family thought that I could re-arrange my lifestyle, to allow for this change in behavior. I call it a change in behavior, because that's what it actually is. It takes a change in your behavior, to fully give up carbs. This change in behavior has been so beneficial for me, that I don't know if I can explain all the benefits here, and still keep this article to less than 2000 words. But I'll try.

**You have to know this!** The biggest benefit I received right off the bat (after about a month), was the weight loss I experienced, that I could not achieve, while I was eating carbs. I not only had lost the 10 lbs I was overweight, I lost another 10 lbs on top of that. I could do things, all of a sudden, that I couldn't do since before my brain injury, 31 years prior. This actually brought about a new life in me. I'm not tired all the time like I use to be. Although I can (and do sometimes), work all day long on an empty stomach, I'm not hungry. Yes I feel the hunger pangs, but they're so easy to ignore, that after a few seconds they disappear, and I don't feel them anymore. That, in my estimation, is the greatest gift this diet has given me. My ability to go hour after hour after hour after hour, sometimes up to 16 hours, if I need to, without eating and most importantly without running out of energy. What a blessing this diet has been for me. Thank you Dr Perlmutter. You'll never believe how much money I save, by not going down the bread aisle at the grocery store, anymore, or the pasta aisle anymore. Staying out of the bakery has probably saved me the most money. I know it's done more to save my life and preserve my health than it's saved me in money, that I would have spent on groceries. The benefit it's been for my health is truly unsurpassable, to say the least.

1. **Weight lifted off my shoulders** This was the feeling I first had when I realized that I was in full control of my weight and henceforth, my health. As I said before, this was the most liberating experience I've ever felt since my coast to coast motorcycle ride. What an exhilarating experience, I hadn't felt that alive, like I said, in 35 years. All of my senses were growing keener, my capabilities were expanding at what felt like an exponential rate. I couldn't believe it. I felt like shouting from the rooftops. I'm not the only one this has happened to. It happened to one of my best friends, who went on a keto diet to help him with his high *PSA* levels, failing kidney functions, deep vein thrombosis and the threat of cancer after having a kidney removed due to a tumor on it. His keto diet had allowed him to drop his medication list from 23 medications to 14, in the first 6 months. He's since dropped his medication list down again to 8 medications. He tells me, he's blowing his doctors and therapists away, because none of them are familiar with the benefits of this diet. He's teaching them.
2. **More Energy** is quite possibly the biggest benefit I've experienced. I honestly know what it's like to run efficiently, on empty. This was a feeling

that was completely foreign to me, prior to my transformation.
I've never been able to keep going, like this before, on an empty stomach.
And I do it day after day after day, never losing energy or stamina. My
energy levels have risen to the extent, that I often work 18 hour days with
few breaks and only one meal, that I nibble on throughout the day. I
seldom have to stop just to eat. I only do so after being reminded, that I
need to put something in my body, to keep it going. I sometimes get,
strange feeling the hunger pangs without feeling hungry. I tell myself to
embrace this feeling, because when this happens, I'm setting my brain up
for future growth. Yes, I said that right,

3.  **Brain growth.** Studies have shown, that the fatter you are the smaller
    your brain is, and it only diminishes in size the fatter you grow. Studies
    have also shown that the thinner you are the larger your brain is, and
    often the exact opposite occurs, the thinner you are, the larger your brain
    grows, allowing you to enjoy the benefits of not only having a larger brain,
    but being able to use it. This has to do with the production of BDNF.
    BDNF, is what sets your brain up to allow it to grow, which you can find
    out more in *Grain Brain*. *"Brain-derived neurotrophic factor, also known
    as BDNF, is a protein that, in humans, is encoded by the
    BDNF gene. BDNF is a member of the neurotrophin family of growth
    factors, which are related to the canonical Nerve Growth
    Factor. Neurotrophic factors are found in the brain and the periphery"*,
    according to Wikipedia. *"BDNF has also demonstrated to increase the
    body's natural antioxidant defenses by boosting enzymes and molecules
    that are important in quenching excessive free radicals"*, as reported by Dr
    Perlmutter. As I mention directly below, the hungrier you can go, the
    more BDNF your body can produce, as calorie restriction increases the
    production of this brain growth protein/antioxidant booster. Not only
    calorie restriction enables its production, but exercise also activates the
    production of this protein, making exercise as important as a good keto
    diet, to allow the body, to maximize the build-up of this protein in your
    system. This is what, initially, allowed our hunter-gatherer ancestors, to
    succeed in the animal world, where other mammals couldn't keep up with
    them, in their evolutionary cycle. By running after game and from being
    preyed on, their exercise worked to build up their brains and mental
    powers. This in return allowed modern man to evolve into what we've
    evolved into, a mammal intelligent enough to build the world we live in
    today and allows us to look into space for the future. Could this BDNF be
    the substance in our bodies, that have allowed our species to advance, to
    the extent we have? With the added brain power I've discovered, I
    shouldn't even have to explain how this is helping my IQ.

4. **Build up of my immune system.** As important as the BDNF, is to brain growth, it's also an important antioxidant, which is what protects our cells from oxidative damage. *NRF2* is another antioxidant, important to cellular protection. *Nrf2* is as important to cellular protection as *BDNF* is to brain growth. *NRF2* is a basic leucine zipper (bZIP) protein that regulates the expression of antioxidant proteins that protect against oxidative damage triggered by injury and inflammation. Several drugs that stimulate the NFE2L2 pathway are being studied for treatment of diseases that are caused by oxidative stress. "Not surprisingly, calorie restriction has been demonstrated in a variety of laboratory animals to induce Nfr2 activation", said Dr Perlmutter in his book *Grain Brain,* meaning the hungrier you can stay, the more you'll build up this important antioxidant protein. And of course, having the ability to increase the amount of this antioxidant in your system, is only going to improve your life, by cutting down on the amount of time you present an illness or disease and that means less trips to your doctor. What more can you ask for? I don't experience headaches anymore, I don't experience colds or the flu as often as I did before, I just don't get sick as much as I used to. Even the mucous in my sinuses has abated, not making me blow my nose as much as I used to. This alone has help cut back on the sinus headaches to the point, to where I only need an aleve for a headache about once every 2 or 3 months. This is something I could never experience while on my high carb diet. Living without as much illness and disease, can save me countless dollars, that I would otherwise waste, just trying to either cure my ailments or even just live with the diseases that I would inevitably have, if I were to remain on a carbohydrate diet. We all know how cheap it is, to not get sick,

5. **Pain Control** could be the next best thing that's happened to me. My pain levels have continuously and steadily abated, from the high levels they were at, when I was eating carbs. This reduction in pain has opened up even more doors for me, as it's easier to exercise harder, giving me a greater benefit from my workouts, not only for my body, but for my brain as well. being able to take advantage of a harder workout allows my body to build greater amounts of BDNF in my system, allowing my system to better regulate the oxidation to my cells that contribute to my pain by not allowing inflammation to infiltrate my body. The inflammation, is caused, directly, by eating a high carbohydrate diet. Cut the Carbs Cut the Inflammation. Cut the medical expense. It's that simple.

6. **Stabilization of Emotions.** This is the most important factor of this diet, as far as everyone who interacts with me on a daily basis knows, I now don't lose my temper as often. I don't get frustrated as often, I don't have

the mood swings that I used to have, from the fluctuations in my blood glucose. That's something that only happens on a high carb diet. On low carb diets, they're virtually non-existent. I often wish that this information had been known 31 years ago. I wonder if it had, would a better diet had enabled me, to speed my healing, 31 years ago? I knew, then, that whole grains were good for me, because it was professed everywhere I went. Even though a good portion of these studies were available for examination at that time, few doctors, specialists, or nutritionists knew of them, because of the suppression of the studies. Who suppressed them and why, is going to take up, probably, multiple articles, to completely untangle that quagmire. The fact remains, that I am much more even tempered now, simply because my blood sugars don't fluctuate, because I have virtually no blood glucose in my system. My system runs on fat and ketones, because fat, is more than 200% more efficient than carbs. Is it any wonder, that you have to eat so many of them, to get just half the energy out of them? My body runs so much better on this "high octane" fuel, that I save money every time I don't go out to eat, because I won't eat what they want to feed me. I have to be very careful when I dine out, and you should too, because restaurants know the cycle that bread puts your through, how it makes you hungry just after you eat it, because of the fluctuations in your blood sugars. That's why they're happy to give you a bread basket, as soon as your seated. They're often taken with the hostess as she seats you, because they know that those rolls, biscuits, bread, or any other of a myriad of sugar de-stabilizers are going to make you order more when your waitress or waiter comes to take it. More than saving money from not eating at restaurants, I save money every time I go to the grocery store, which actually, I'm visiting much less these days (and that saves me even more money). But this point begs the question, who shelved these studies, so the medical community and even more importantly, the FDA and ADA, who structure our food guidelines, that tell us what's healthy to eat and what's not, couldn't even look at the data? Why didn't they deem this information that important? Could it have been the involvement of the crop seed companies, who sell their crop seed to farmers to grow it? Could it have been the grain industry? Could it have been the restaurant industry? Could it have been the bread industry?

7. **Liberation From Corporate Control** This will probably be the most important aspect of this diet, in my life, going forward. The freedom I'm able to experience, because I'm not a slave to those pesky carbs, has more to do with corporate control than most of you want to realize. By controlling the amount of sugar they put in your diet, they control your

buying habits. Who hasn't been addicted to chocolate? The reason they addict you to chocolate is, so you'll buy more. They do it with chocolate, they do it with all candies, all breads, all pastas, all cereals, all forms of alcohol, even all juices and soft drinks, they want you addicted to this huge cash cow, because that's the nature of the business they're in. They make a consumable product, that's so sweet and tasty, people everywhere love it and buy it, and they don't even have to put anything extra in it to make it addictive, because it already is, due to its massive sugar content. This is the control that, these industries are imposing on those willing to fall for this ruse. What are their motives? Is their motivation little more than greed? They have to know, how they're feeding the obesity epidemic, which feeds the diabetes epidemic, which feeds the dementia epidemic and also feeds the cancer epidemic, the cardio-vascular epidemic, the arthritis epidemic, the gastro-intestinal epidemic, the headache (migraine, sinus and stress) epidemic, and the Celiac disease that exists in the thousands of us? They obviously feed this food to their families, because they get just as sick as the rest of those who remain on a carb diet. This tells me that they don't know what they're forcing the world to live on and with, due to the consequences of living on it, themselves. I honestly think that all farmers, think that they are serving the world a purpose by growing this grain, for us. I honestly don't believe that they know just how dangerous it really is. They can't, and still grow it. So it must be, that they're being lied to, to continue to grow it. After all this is what keep the money coming in.

8. **Freedom From Illness and Disease** I know I touched on this before, in point 4 when I talked about the tremendous boost my in immune system, but I have to re-iterate how much benefit this one factor alone, has granted me. Not getting sick has to be the single best thing I can do for my body. It frees up so much time, that it's not even funny. Not getting sick allows me to always be at the gym every day I need to go. This allows me to build up that BDNF, that's so important in helping me to expand my mental capabilities. It also help me to reinforce my auto-immune system, by building this same protein along with the Nrf2 that also builds up my anti-oxidants. These two gems allow me to stay healthier, keeping me clear of the doctor's office, except for routine wellness visits. The savings in money not spent is quite substantial. The fact of the matter is, that I already have too much wrong with me for anything else to go awry. I can't afford to aggravate the problems I still have, the high blood pressure (even though I control it with my keto diet), chronic pain, hemiplegia, severe BPH (due to medications I was on for over 12 years), that all began with the severe closed head injury that I've

learned to deal with, for 31 years. With all of these "pre-existing" conditions, left over from when I was on a carb diet, I can't afford to acquire any more. The beauty is, I'm continuing to diminish my afflictions, instead of aggravating them, simply because of my MCT keto diet. One of the biggest improvements I had right off the bat, was the end to the acid indigestion, stomach cramps, and headaches. All of these were manifestations of the wheat I was eating. But they've been gone for so long now, that I forgot all about them.

A few more words to express the wonders that this diet has brought to my body, should be set forth here, before I close out this edition of this series. In my life, I've never had as much energy as what I do right now. I just got my blood work back earlier this week and after discussing my diet with my doctor, to make sure, everything I'm doing is safe and productive. All my blood tests have come back with results like I've never seen before. My high blood pressure is a thing of the past. My cholesterol levels, although being high (which is what I want), are better balanced than they've ever been in my entire life (high HDL, low LDL and VLDL). All of the panels requested, in my blood work, were as normal as they've ever been. My doctor aid, after seeing my results from my blood work, " whatever you're doing, is good. Keep it up."

I still have high blood pressure because I've been diagnosed with it in the past, I'm just controlling it with my diet. How easy this control, is! When my blood pressure was checked the other afternoon around 3PM (when your blood pressure is often the highest), it was 120/60, which is the benchmark of normal blood pressure. You just can't get results this good on a carbohydrate diet. They're only possible on a low carb diet. They're even more possible on a MCT ketogenic diet like the one I'm currently on. If this kind of a diet could to this for me, with all the health problems that I've had, can you imagine what it could do for you? The only way you'll know, is if you try it out. I can make you this guarantee, that you will experience most all of the same benefits, that I've experienced, if you were to transform your diet into a high fat, low carb diet. Anyway you look at it, it's a win, win, win situation, for anybody who has the courage to accomplish it. One month is all you need to see results.

**GO CARB FREE,**

**EXPERIENCE THE FREEDOM**

**THAT THE CARB FREE FEW**

**ALREADY KNOW.**

# ARTICLE 18
# WEIGHT LOSS - OVSERVATIONS FROM MY OWN JOURNEY IN ABSTAINING FROM WHEAT

Eight years and 60 lbs ago, I decided after looking at my driver's license picture, that I had to make some changes in the form of weight loss or I was going to die much sooner than I had planned to. I knew that I had to get back to where I used to be, twenty years earlier, when I weighed 155lbs. It seems that all of a sudden, I turned into a very "cheeky fellow". I mean that my cheeks looked like they belonged to chipmunks. Problem was, they had nothing in them...except fat. I had become very comfortable eating every kind of pastry, pasta and bread that I could find, thinking that it was all healthy for me and wasn't affecting my weight in the slightest. Boy was I wrong!

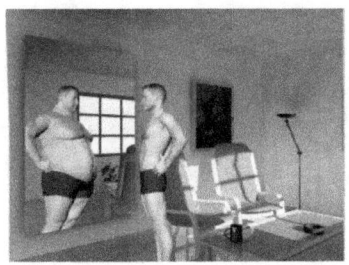

Fortunately for me, a farmer's market opened up by me, that carried a lot of bulk foods. This allowed me to cut down or even stop eating processed foods and concentrate more on preparing everything for myself. I soon learned the best way to lose weight for me was to limit my intake of breads (which I love) and grain based snack foods and eat more fruits and vegetables, not only for meals but for snacks between meals.

I'm one of those, now, that believes that fruits and vegetables should be at the bottom of the old food pyramid that I followed growing up. instead of grains because it's the fruits and vegetables that are really the most nutritious. Now don't get me wrong. I didn't say to stop eating breads, I'm just saying that you should limit your intake. But I am saying that you should stop eating all snacks made out of grains, especially wheat. (*That was when I wrote this in 2013.* I've since learned better and changed my mind.)

Roy Knight Jr

For me, the ratio was directly proportional, the more fruit and vegetables I ate, the more weight I lost. The more breads and snacks I ate, the more weight I gained. For me it was easy, just cut out all the breads and snacks and eat only fruits and vegetables.

That worked until I became anemic and had to start taking B-12 tablets. That was when I decided to put meat back into my diet and with meat came the grains in the form of breads, pastas, and cereals. After the meat and grains came the weight. I say this to point out the fact that balance is what's most important, for when I became anemic, I was 10 lbs under my optimal weight after losing close to 50 lbs. I lost it by eating nothing but fruits and vegetables and in doing that I lost the balance. I may have lost some weight but I lost some of my health also.

Now I make sure that I have more meat in my diet by having at least one serving each day and I try to control the amount of breads, pastas and cereals so I can maintain a weight that's optimal for me. But then, even though exercise has always been a part of my daily routine, it's the food side of the equation that I'm dwelling on with this article.

Balance is the optimal expression here. We just need to make sure that our balance should tip to the fruit and vegetable side of the plate. Changing snack food to fruits and nuts instead of grain products like pastries and cookies might be the most important change that I've made. Although I haven't tried the Fat Burning Brownies or the Guilt Free Chocolate yet, I'm almost sorry to say that I never will as I have learned that there's something to the claim that Dr William Davis made in his book Wheat Belly, because I've broke my addiction to breads and pastas and I've dropped another 5 lbs. Best thing yet? It's still off after 1 month, so I would highly recommend that you read Wheat Belly by Dr William Davis. It's an eye opening book in which Dr Davis claims that wheat should be called "Frankenwheat" due to it addictive nature as well as the lack of nutrition that it now has due to genetic engineering, simply to get more crop out of an acre of ground. I said goodbye to wheat. You should try if you think you can? Because of it's addictive nature, I can guarantee you that it'll be tougher than you think, but the rewards for doing so far outweigh the consequences of not doing so.

After trying to eliminate all wheat from my diet, I was able to eliminate 98% of it. Not until trying to eliminate it all did I ever realize how prevalent it is in our daily diet. It's no wonder we're so overweight. Wheat products are everywhere you turn in the grocery store. Every restaurant serves some form of it. It's the next thing closest to impossible to get away from. But since trying to do exactly that 1 month ago, I've lost another 5 lbs. to where I'm only 5 lbs away from my optimum weight for my height, with my BMI being 1/10th of a point from being excellent (20.1) for my age. I had an idea that it was the breads that wasn't letting me get past the point I was at, but I had little idea how much they were hindering me. Since I've all but stopped them completely, my moods have stabilized and I'm not so quick to anger, probably because my blood sugars are staying on a more even level. I've replaced the breads with more nutritious foods (fruits and vegetables) which have far more micro-nutrients in them than what the bread has. This one little change has perhaps had more influence on my life and interaction with people than almost anything else. Breads weren't just hurting my body, but they were hurting my brain as well.

I'm doing my best to stay off the grain products and it's going good except for a few crackers once in a while. If I'm not careful though, my old addiction will kick in and I'll end up gorging out on not just crackers, but any or all grain products like pastries, pasta, and bread as well as the worst of them all, cookies and donuts. There's so many of them out there and there so easy to consume, it's like it's a conspiracy to keep me eating that which is least healthiest for me. I almost feel like a rebel trying to break away from this crap but this is something I feel good about rebelling against. After falling back to my old addiction and increasing my bread intake, I managed to put on 5 lbs. but fortunately, taking it back off was as easy as stopping the grain intake, because it came right back off within a week after I cut back. Since then, I've stayed off of it, and managed to lose another 3 lbs. I'm now within 2 lbs of my target weight. This was a weight I never thought I could achieve and I'm only 2 lbs away bringing me to this conclusion, grain products offer too little nourishment for the amount of weight gain they bring. They're too heavy on the simple starches that add weight and too light on the complex carbohydrates that have the micro-nutrients that give me the nutrition I need. This throws the balance too far away from healthy for me.

141

Roy Knight Jr

It's been about 3 months since I decided to quit eating bread products, for all intents and purposes. But it's impossible to do away with altogether. I see now how this could be the biggest crisis to America, since the Cold War, the assumption that bread products of all kinds are somehow good for us. Since I cut back on my intake of bread three months ago, I've lost another 12 lbs and am now below my ideal weight by 2 lbs. The beauty of it is, I know my weight is going to stay here as long as I control the amount of bread products that I put in my mouth to eat. The fewer grain products I eat the easier it is to lose weight. If I want to maintain my weight I include a little bit of them in my diet. If I want to lose weight I eat less grains (breads, cakes, pastries, danish, pasta, noodles, rice & rice dishes, cereal, granola, popcorn, etc). I have to admit that going without eating all of the products listed is the next thing closest to impossible, but if I control the intake of those products, I control my weight.

This is to the point where it's almost unbelievable except for the fact that I'm living it. And experiencing it! 4 Months and counting, with reduced grains and **no wheat**.  An additional 18 lbs and holding. My weight is at a 27 year low. The last time it was this low, I was recovering from being in a coma for a month. This weight loss that I've experienced just from cutting back on grains and eliminating wheat and anything that contains any portion of wheat, has manifested multiple other blessings on my body, brain and behavior. One of the biggest blessings is I'm not hungry all of the time. It's becoming almost too easy to ignore my stomach, which is something I've never been able to do. That's alright because now I can eat more than I ever used to eat and I still lose weight.  Although I may be to my ideal weight now, as my weight has stayed the same for about a week.  The benefits though don't stop with my reduced weight. They go much farther than that. I don't feel the pain of arthritis as much, my stomach doesn't act up as much, my thinking is much, much clearer. That's probably due to the more stable glucose levels in my blood. This book, Wheat Belly, has truly changed my life. If you were smart, you'd let it change yours too.

In my continuing chronicle of my abstinence from wheat, it's been about 4 1/2 months, my weight has hit a 28 year low and I've been accused of turning skinny. It may be time to reintroduce wheat back into my diet and I would except for the few times that I've tried it already. When I did add wheat

142

back into my diet, problems started to arise that essentially reminded me of why it was such a good idea to quit, such as my joints would start hurting again, I'd start itching usually about 5-10 minutes after I ingested the bread or cracker. So now that I've found out that I indeed do have an intolerance to wheat, I'm in the search for products of this nature that won't contain any wheat within them. This is a challenge that I didn't expect to run into, finding breads and crackers that don't have any wheat flour contained within them. I know enough to look for gluten free products but half of the problem is that the fillers they use for the gluten are more fattening than the gluten itself. But it's not just the gluten that bothers me, it's the gliadin, the part responsible for aggravating any arthritis you might have in your body as well as damaging your brain cells beyond repair. It turns out then, that it seems to be a really good idea to give up the wheat products for more reasons than just the weight loss. By quitting the wheat, I'm saving my brain as well as my body. I would have never guessed that in a million years, that such a simple product as bread or pasta, could cause so many problems in our bodies or our brains. My next read is to learn more precisely what grains in general are doing to our brains by reading Grain Brain by Dr Perlmutter.

I'm now about 6 months into my new life without wheat or now, without any grains. After reading Grain Brain, all carbohydrates have been reduced, in my diet, with the exception of green vegetables and fruits in limited amounts. My weight is hovering around 15 lbs lower than my ultimate dream weight, a weight that I never thought I could achieve. It's amazing how just giving up one kind of food source could have such an impact on one's health. It's amazing how much better life is overall now. The arthritis that's plagued my back for 30 years has reduced in severity to less than half as bad as it was when I was eating them. I'm doing things I haven't been able to do for more than 30 years. My thinking is clearer. My emotions have evened out from not having the highs and lows from changes in my blood glucose. It's almost unbelievable how much better I feel...and all from eating no more grains. What a Deal!! And I thought Wheat Belly changed my life. That impact is insignificant compared to what I've learned from Grain Brain.

Two weeks later and I'm still losing weight, to the point that I'm at the lowest weight I've seen in 30 years. My total weight loss is now over 60 lbs and again I'm being accused of being too skinny. I remember being accused of that in high school. All of this is the result of a high fat, low or no carb diet. I have to admit that it wasn't easy but it was well worth it and after I broke the addiction of the wheat and grains, the pounds kept melting off effortlessly. And now that I've been off of them for 6 months, I can't go back to eating them, for all the problems that they create, so I'm pretty much guaranteed that I'm not going to put the weight back on.

This is the really interesting part, according to Dr Perlmutter in his book, Grain Brain, your body creates certain hormones that strengthen and build your brain when you're thinner and when you fast without food. This seems to be the case for me as it's much easier to finish my crossword puzzles now. What a deal...weight loss combined with loss of arthritis and a more balanced emotional state and best of all a lot more brain power. I couldn't have bargained for anything better.

4 months later and my weight seems to have leveled out at 55 pounds lower than it was at my heaviest, 210 lbs. For the last 3 months my weight has been right around 155lbs, which is exactly 10 lbs heavier than when I was 28yrs old. Since adapting a high fat, lo - no carb diet, I can't seem to put on weight, even though I'm eating more. Maybe it just seems like I'm eating more because I'm eating more often, sometimes 6 times a day. I'm still adjusting to how easy it is to do everything again. Little things like getting up and down have become so easy again, I can either sit on the floor or stand up from the floor without the use of my arms or hands and if that doesn't sound like too much, you should try it sometime. It's something I haven't been able to do for over 30 years. My arthritis has diminished tremendously to where many of the pains are just nuisance pains. My stomach never gets upset anymore and I don't seem to get headaches anymore. It's turned out that this decision to quit eating cereal grains has been the healthiest decision I've ever made.

8 months and I bet you're all waiting to see if I've put back on my weight or not. You want to see if this change is permanent or not. My weight has increased back to 160 lbs, but I'm eating a lot more since I've been finding more and more foods to eat that don't have any grains in them and since my weight is still 15 lbs below what my weight should be for my height, I'm quite happy staying slender. I actually have a "sculpted body" now. I've never had

a sculpted body. Even when I was 28 and had a somewhat sculpted body, my legs were too skinny because I couldn't get over 154 lbs in all my attempts to gain weight. It wasn't until I turned 35 that my weight started to climb. By the time I was 40 it had reached 190 lbs and hit 210 lbs when I turned 53 so needless to say it feels so good to be back down to my normal weight, 160. I just wish I could have had this body when I was 28. The legs may be a little thin yet, but there not skinny.

As far as my other health is concerned, my arthritis has cleared up, I don't have any stomach problems anymore and my thinking is as clear as it's ever been. This abstinence from grains has taught me that grains truly are dangerous foods for the human body.

It's now been close to a year since my decision to quit wheat and grains, and with the exception of my lower back where there exists degenerative disc disease, my health hasn't been better and my weight has stayed at 160 lbs. For my height, that is 15 lbs below my optimum weight, but I'm feeling much better keeping it lower. It's a lot easier to get up and down now, almost as easy as when I was a kid. From a weight of 210 lbs 7 years ago, to 184 a year ago to 160 now, it's become apparent that the true key to weight loss was the disappearance of wheat and grains from my diet. It's also a lot more fun to eat fat again.

Close to 2 years have passed since I originally gave up the grain. I've stayed off the grains but my diet has incorporated more fat to compensate for the loss in calories from the high carbohydrate grains. I've even taken to taking a sip of coconut oil every once in a while, simply because it tastes good. My weight fluctuates now, between 155 and 160, usually staying closer to 155 most of the time. There are times, however, when I eat too much and when I do that my weight goes up simply because of the amount of food I ate. But then, it always drops back down the next day. It feels so much better being at a weight that I was trying to achieve 35 years ago when I was in my mid-twenties. Back then, I was trying to gain weight, because everybody considered me skinny. After I hit 35, the weight really came on, so much so, that I couldn't get it back off. Not until I gave up what was keeping that weight on me, the high carbohydrate foods, that are mostly found in grain foods, like bread, cereal, pasta and pastries. High carbohydrate food includes foods with sugar and sweeteners in them, as well as sodas, fruit drinks and alcohol. New studies have shown that diet sodas don't help anyone keep their weight down. The artificial sweeteners, it seems, trick the body into wanting more, which can be deadly, if you're already overweight.

**I learned that eating fat, doesn't make you fat. What makes you fat is eating carbs.**

It all has to do with the way your body metabolizes carbs. You can know this by reading Grain Brain by Dr David Perlmutter, or Wheat Belly by Dr William Davis. They'll both tell you just how devastating this food source can be. And it can be pretty devastating.

After I learned that 1 gram of glucose, (the fuel of carbs) has 4 calories, as opposed to the 9 calories of fuel in each gram of fat, it occurred to me that fat is a much more efficient fuel than the glucose is. That means that you don't have to eat nearly as much, if you're on a diet that uses healthy fats and protein instead of a diet that uses  high carbohydrate food. Actually you can get all the nutrition out of half the amount of high fat foods as what you get out of a high carbohydrate food. I've been told that the diet I'm on now is actually a ketogenic diet. Ketogenic diets are usually used for people fighting illness or disease. What I've really learned is that Ketogenic diets are for healthy people and anybody who wants to be healthy, because our bodies, genetically, have not advanced enough through evolution to handle the extreme load of glucose that carbs put into the body. I've learned that carbs, especially too many of them can be deadly, simply because of  amount of illness and disease they cause, like diabetes, arthritis, cancer, high blood pressure, heart disease, and too many more that room prohibits me from listing them.

Suffice it to say, carbs are bad food to eat. If you switch to a Ketogenic diet and allow your body to go into ketosis, you'll find that your energy reserves rise dramatically, as well as a return to your previous healthy state when you were younger. For me, it was 40 years younger. You should try it. I can absolutely guarantee that you will like it.

Now, it's been 28 months since I've gone "carb free" and what a trip its been. My weight is still 154 right now. sometimes it fluctuates up to 156 or down to 152, but it's always in that range, 20+ lbs lower than my prescribed weight. My pain is reduced. The inflammation throughout my entire body is reduced. My headaches are non-existent. I have less mucus in my sinuses. I sweat less because of the lack of fat on my body. My arthritis doesn't bother me nearly as much. I don't have stomach problems anymore, ever. Most importantly, I have more energy, a lot more energy and I'm not hungry half the time. When I am hungry, it's easy to ignore. This is true bliss. My blood pressure last time I checked it, was 115/60. It's never been that low. It's always been in the 130/80 range to 140 /90 range, while at rest. This lack of carbs in my diet has lowered my blood pressure, lowered my blood glucose, balanced my cholesterol, (To those uneducated about cholesterol, I lowered my LDL Cholesterol that's the bad stuff.) To learn exactly what this transformation has done to my life, visit *Carbs, My Life Without Them.*

With fat being 225% more efficient than carbs, why would anyone in their right mind ever return to carbs? I love eating fat, to not be fat.

One thing I refuse to do, is to give in to the food/pharmaceutical industrial complex. I will not play their game and fall into their trap, the trap of eating their food, then having to buy their drugs to cure the illness their food causes. My mama didn't raise a sucker.

Less than two months later on 3/20/16, my book has been published for two weeks. I have 3 proofs with another 2 on the way. *It's Time For A Cure* is available in color, and *Its' Time To Curb Your Carbs to Save Your Life And Keep Your Dignity*

By April 28, 1016 my book has been published for 5 weeks, I have given out about 8-10 copies to acquaintances and friends and church members, and have received excellent reviews so far.

Final update on May4, 2016. My ketogenic diet has improved my health in unimaginable ways. From fewer mosquito bites to less grey hair, the changes have been phenomenal.

# ARTICLE 19
# THE GLYCEMIC INDEX; YOUR GUIDE TO HEALTH

Now that we know what this food staple has been doing for us as well as what it's doing to us, how is this information going to help us, if we don't know what kind of foods they're actually coming from. That's what we're going to talk about here. What should I eat? What effect will this have on my body? What shouldn't I eat and what effect will that have on my body?

Before we can start on the foods that at good for us and the ones that aren't, we have to talk about the effect these foods have on the Glycemic Index, and how that impacts what effect they have on your body. First thing you should know is that foods that are lower on the glycemic index are much healthier than those that are higher on the index.

This is due to the amount of sugars that are present in the food, that influence your blood glucose, making necessary the production of insulin in your body. Insulin is what you need to digest carbohydrates, to turn them into a fuel that your body can use, fat. The higher the food is on the glycemic index, the more insulin it needs to be digested and hence because it need more insulin, that means it going to create more fat. This is your body's Fat Factory and it's carbohydrates, that turn it on. This is how it works.

It's the insulin that turns carbohydrates into fat, so they can be burned and used by the body. The more carbohydrates you feed yourself, the more sugar you're feeding the Fat Factory and the more glucose you're pouring into your system, requiring your pancreas to crank out more insulin to digest those carbohydrates. Because, carbs aren't fully digested in your intestines, they're simply broken down into sugars to be metabolized cellularly with insulin. The more glucose you have in your system, the more insulin your body needs to turn all that glucose into fat. The more insulin you need to digest your carbs, year after year, the more this puts your pancreas into a mode that keeps generating insulin and after a while your body becomes adjusted to the excessive amounts of insulin in your system to digest the excessive amounts of carbs in your system and you body becomes insulin resistant. This is type 2 diabetes and it's deadly. This is what leads to four of the deadliest of cancers, most of all cardiovascular diseases (which are the number one killer or all diseases), all Alzheimer's disease as well as most all brain disorders. It also plays a major role in many emotional disorders. This is why it's so important to control the intake of sugars into your body and carbohydrates are sugars.

## So, what should we be eating and what shouldn't we be eating?

Starchy carbs are the foods that occupy the highest slots on the glycemic index, with the exception of alcohol and beer, and potatoes and parsnips which are also very high on the index. Beer is one of two things that can raise your blood sugar more than pure glucose, which is what the index is based on.

According to Wikipedia: "The glycemic index or glycaemic index (GI) is a number associated with a particular type of food that indicates the food's effect on a person's blood glucose (also called blood sugar) level. A value of 100 represents the standard, an equivalent amount of pure glucose."

"The GI represents the total rise in a person's blood sugar level following consumption of the food; it may or may not represent the rapidity of the rise in blood sugar. The steepness of the rise can be influenced by a number of other factors, such as the quantity of fat eaten with the food. The GI is useful for understanding how the body breaks down carbohydrates and only takes into account the available carbohydrate (total carbohydrate minus fiber) in a food. Although the food may contain fats and other components that contribute to the total rise in blood sugar, these effects are not reflected in the GI."

"The glycemic index is usually applied in the context of the quantity of the food and the amount of carbohydrate in the food that is actually consumed. A related measure, the glycemic load (GL), factors this in by multiplying the glycemic index of the food in question by the carbohydrate content of the actual serving. Watermelon has a high glycemic index, but a low glycemic load for the quantity typically consumed. Fructose, by contrast, has a low glycemic index, but can have a high glycemic load if a large quantity is consumed."

"Glycemic load is based on the glycemic index (GI), and is calculated by multiplying the grams of available carbohydrate in the food times the food's GI and then dividing by 100. Glycemic load estimates the impact of carbohydrate consumption using the glycemic index while taking into account the amount of carbohydrate that is consumed. GL is a GI-weighted measure of carbohydrate content. For instance, watermelon has a high GI, but a typical serving of watermelon does not contain much carbohydrate, so the glycemic load of eating it is low. Whereas glycemic index is defined for each type of food, glycemic load can be calculated for any size serving of a food, an entire meal, or an entire day's meals."

The above 4 paragraphs were taken from Wikipedia for a reason, as important as the glycemic index is, it's the glycemic load that's more important, because this is what dictates how much insulin your body is going to need to digest all the carbohydrates you eat. It also tells you how much fat that food is going to create when you eat it. The only thing that creates fat in your body is carbohydrates and how much they create, can be seen by how high a food is on the glycemic index and what load it carries. The higher a food is on the glycemic index, the more fattening it is. The more glycemic load it carries, the more fat it creates. It's that simple.

If it's glucose in the system that leads to fat on the body, what does that tell us? To stay away from foods that raise the glucose levels in your blood. When you look at all the foods on the glycemic index, you'll see all the starchy foods that are grain based, at the higher levels of the glycemic index. This one factor should tell you to stay away from those foods. Problem is, those foods are the ones that are most addictive, simply because of the amount of sugar (carbs) in them.

The first thing you need to recognize is that carbohydrates are not nutrition, by themselves. They simply offer a path to get that nutrition into your body. Carbohydrates are complex sugars that are turned into fat, the kind of fat, your body doesn't use that much. We may have used that fat in the past, but we don't anymore, due to our sedentary lifestyle.

When you eat fruits and vegetables, you're eating carbohydrates, but the trade off of the nutrition you're getting with the small amount of sugar that comes with it, makes it worth the trade off. These sugars are absorbed much slower so they don't spend as much time floating around in the blood waiting for insulin to be turned into fat. (This is when sugar is at its most dangerous point, waiting for something to cling onto, whether it be insulin, or fat or protein, either of which end up becoming glycated into plaque and inflammation.) This is not what the body needs. But the sugars are tied up with fiber (in the more complex carbohydrates), so they're not absorbed as quick as simpler sugars…the kind that come with grains.

That means you need to weigh the nutrition you're getting from the food against the number of empty starchy carbs that you're putting into that same system. Does this food offer enough nutrition for all the sugar you're getting out of it? If so, is it worth the tradeoff?

This is where grain based foods fall short. **None** of them have enough nutrition to counterbalance the amount of carbs they put into your system. The sugar overload is just too much. This is because of their easily digestible fiberless carbohydrates that are made from flour and sugar. Despite what others say, any food that's made out of whole wheat has hardly any fiber that's worth anything. What fiber it had, was lost as soon as it was milled into flour and it's the flour that you need to make any bread product, like pastries, pasta, cereals, tortillas, crackers, cookies, cakes. Without milling the flour, the grain can't be used to make any of the comfort foods that everyone loves to eat so much. This is what makes the food so satiating or satisfying, the amount of sugar it immediately dumps into your body to create more fat. This is also what makes it so dangerous as well as addictive, but then, you know that by now. I can only hope that you've discovered ideas of how to eliminate this from your diet, from reading *Carbs, How To Cut Back.*

Quite possibly the most important carbs to avoid are the ones you drink. The ones that come from sodas, fruit drinks and juices and worst of all alcohol, grain alcohol should be avoided at all costs. Rule # 1 when it comes to cutting your carbs, is to stop drinking your calories. Those calories are truly worthless calories and should be the first to be removed from your diet.

Too often though, these carbs are the most addictive making them the hardest to stop. We all know how addictive alcohol is. Where does most drinkable alcohol come from? Carbohydrates, like fruit and grains. Both make ethanol, ethyl alcohol, which is the predominant alcohol in alcoholic beverages" This means that they are concentrated sugars, waiting to create fat in your Fat Factory. Obviously, this is a whole other world to the sins of sugar. That's why drinking your calories, should be at the top of your NOT TO DO list.

What to do? If you have to have something sweet, don't use artificial sweeteners, as many of those are more fattening that sugar itself or they carry implications of causing cancer. I use Stevia. It's natural and it's very sweet. Too much of it though, can be bitter. As well as being completely natural, it has 0 calories, nor is it linked to cancer in any way, shape or form. I sweeten my green tea with it. (I still haven't been able to drink my tea without it or lemon juice.) I also sweeten my hot chocolate with it.

Even though cheese is stocked by the meat department in most stores, it's actually a dairy product. Cheese comes from milk. I can see where that might raise concerns for someone who is lactose intolerant, but ripened cheeses like Cheddar contain only about 5% of the lactose found in whole milk, and aged cheeses contain almost none, as "Cheese is often avoided by those who are lactose intolerant, but ripened cheeses like Cheddar contain only about 5% of the lactose found in whole milk, and aged cheeses contain almost none."

Nevertheless, people with severe lactose intolerance should avoid eating dairy cheese. As a natural product, the same kind of cheese may contain different amounts of lactose on different occasions, causing unexpected painful reactions. Yet, I had a friend who was lactose intolerant and loved to eat cheese. According to Wikipedia, "For a few cheeses, the milk is curdled by adding acids such as vinegar or lemon juice. Most cheeses are acidified to a lesser degree by bacteria, which turn milk sugars into lactic acid, then the addition of rennet completes the curdling."

Dr Davis has a number of lactose intolerant patients who were cured simply by ending their wheat ingestion. What was thought to be lactose intolerance was actually gluten intolerance. Because once the gluten was removed from the diet, lactose could be re-introduced again back into the diet with no severe reactions. No doctor, at the time though, thought that something made from a staple food such as bread could ever cause something so bad. I guess they never read any of the studies.

What I eat most of myself, are raw nuts. They're super high in clean protein and fats making them very nutritious calories that I use to fuel my body. I say clean protein, because wheat has protein also, but it's not clean. It's a very dirty protein, as it comes with carbohydrates and carbohydrates are the bane of healthy protein because they have a tendency to bend the protein into misshaped amyloids, which are the basis of the deadliest of diseases, both cancer and heart disease. And that's not to mention what it does to the brain. Amyloid plaque is associated with half of the cancers and Atheroma plaque is the biggest player in cardiovascular diseases. And these are only two of the 4 different kinds of plaque caused by this food. That, to me is the definition of dirty protein, especially when you look at what it does to the body.

When people ask me, what exactly do I eat? I say everything, but grains and high starch foods, which actually includes more than grains. It includes potatoes, parsnips and even sweet potatoes. It doesn't include yams, though. They're tubers and have a lot more fiber than potatoes and sweet potatoes, making them much more difficult to digest quickly. Because of their fiber, they're actually digested slowly making their glycemic load much lower than their glycemic index number which is still low.

When I stopped my bread ingestion, I replaced those lost calories in my diet with a lot of yams. They're high in beta-carotene and they taste great. I got in the habit of carrying a baked yam with me, just so I had it to gnaw on, whenever I was hungry.

You basically can't go wrong eating those truly high fiber carbohydrates. Almost all vegetables are excellent sources of nutrition. The nutrition to carb ratio is worth the trade off because the carbs are so slow to digest, lessening their impact on the blood glucose. I say almost, because some vegetables are primarily starch and have little nutritional benefit for the body.

If you're not a vegetarian, meats are excellent sources of clean protein, as most meats have more iron in them than other sources of protein. Eggs are another excellent source of protein and vitamins and minerals, all essential to your health. Dr Perlmutter likes to remind us of the old egg commercials of the *Incredible, Edible Egg*. I still remember the jingle. Eggs are an excellent source of protein and cholesterol. Remember, cholesterol is your friend. Your brain uses cholesterol. Your body uses cholesterol. Your immune system uses cholesterol. There are only a few parts of your body where it isn't important.

What should you fear while choosing your foods? Fear the substance that glycates cholesterol, glucose. It's glucose in the system that gums it up and keeps it from running efficiently. You might find after you cease you intake of wheat and grain products that your options to eat other foods that used to be off limits to you, may be more easier digested. It's happened for a lot of other people, who's to say it can't happen to you?

IT'S YOUR CHOICE TO LIVE WITH PAIN

OR TO LIVE PAINFREE,

TO LIVE WITH DIGESTIVE DISORDERS,

HEART DISEASE,

CANCER AND

ALZHEIMER'S DISEASE

OR BE FREE!

IT'S YOUR CHOICE TO CURE YOURSELF

BY CURBING YOUR CARBS

# ARTICLE 20
# THE POWER OF BEING THIN
# IS FOUND BY EATING FAT

Most everybody wants to be thin simply to look good, but the advantages of being thin go a lot further than just looking good. Being thin is not only highly beneficial for your looks but it's crucial for your health and even more important for your brain's healthy function. Did you know that the fatter you are, the smaller your brain is? It's true. That is directly from Dr Perlmutter's book *Grain Brain.* Conversely, the thinner you are, the bigger your brain is, also. Don't believe me? Look at the research studies and what Dr Perlmutter says in *Grain Brain:*

"The dots connecting excessive body fat, obesity, and brain dysfunction are not hard to follow given the information you've already learned in this book. Excessive body fat increases not only insulin resistance, but also the production of inflammatory chemicals that play directly into brain degeneration. For this very reason, waist circumference is often a measurement of "health," as it predicts future health challenges and mortality; the higher your waist circumference, the higher your risk for disease and death."

"It's well documented that visceral fat is uniquely capable of triggering inflammatory pathways in the body as well as signaling molecules that disrupt the body's normal course of hormonal actions. In addition, visceral fat does more than just generate inflammation down the road through a chain of biological events; visceral fat itself becomes inflamed. This kind of fat houses tribes of inflammatory white blood cells. In fact, the hormonal and inflammatory molecules produced by visceral fat get dumped directly into the liver, which, as you can imagine, responds with another round of ammunition (i.e., inflammatory reactions and hormone-disrupting substances). Long story short: More than merely a predator lurking behind a tree, it is an enemy that is armed and dangerous. The number of health conditions now linked to visceral fat is tremendous, from the obvious ones such as obesity and metabolic syndrome to the not-so-obvious—cancer, autoimmune disorders, and brain disease."

I copied the information above from *Grain Brain* for a reason. Obesity is a danger to more than just your body, It's shrinking your brain by eating it up slowly and it's all due to excessive carbohydrate consumption, carbohydrates in the form of cereals, breads and pastas. It's true, according to Donald W. Miller, Jr., MD, "Carbohydrates are the primary cause of weight gain, not fats. (Animals raised for food are fattened with carbohydrates.)" He goes on to say that "eating fat is not only healthier than eating carbohydrates, it makes you thinner." Yes, it's true, eating fat makes you thin.

**Eat Fat To Be Thin**

I know that sounds strange, but I'll explain, since you body runs on fat, not sugar, it only makes sense to feed it what it wants, healthy fat to burn. When you feed your body health fats, it doesn't have to make changes to that food before it can use it as it's ready to use. That means that it doesn't get stored, like fat from carbohydrates.

Carbohydrates have always been nothing more than an emergency basis food, this is food we eat when we can't find healthy fat and protein. Evolution gave our bodies the ability to digest carbs for those times when we couldn't catch or kill game. Studies have shown that getting back to what our original metabolism likes for a diet and what our bodies are meant to digest means getting back to diet high in fats and low in carbohydrates. **Dr Atkins was the first to promote a low carbohydrate diet as early as 1958**, yet it seems that the carbohydrate addiction complex had already started its devious work in addicting our society to the ravages of the *Wheat Belly* saga. It seems that too many of our congress thought it better to restrict our consumption fats, thinking that's what was causing all the problem with obesity and diabetes. In all actuality, it's carbs that cause the fat that causes obesity and diabetes, not fat at all.

It's all a matter of how they are digested. To digest carbohydrates, your body has to turn them into fat. This is because your body can't run on sugar. It runs on fat. The studies showing this include, Iris Shai, R.D.,Phd (July 2008). "Weight Loss with a Low Carbohydrate, Mediterranean, or Low-Fat Diet" New England Journal of  Medicine 359 (3): 22941. doi:10.1056 /NEJM oa0708681.PMID 18635428, **Low-carbohydrate-Diet Score and the Risk of Coronary Heart Disease in Women from The New England Journal of Medicine**. What this means is that when you eat carbohydrates, your body can't use that as food because it burns fat.

When you eat fat, your body doesn't have to convert that into anything to use. They're digested in your small intestine unlike carbs that are metabolized cellularly with the help of insulin. That means that the glucose that carbs become, have to float around in your blood stream until they can enter a cell, to be used as glycogen. This is where the problem begins. Anyone who's been on a diet of carbohydrates for any amount of time has enough glycogen built up in their systems that they don't need anymore, so the glucose turns into fat to be stored for future use.

The first place your body stores this fat is around your mid section, hence its name, belly fat or visceral fat. This is a dangerous fat to have in your body as this is where diabetes starts, along with a host of cancers and CVDs or heart diseases and most every kind of dementia, including Alzheimer's Disease, Parkinson's Disease and Huntington's Disease. Human biology hasn't changed evolutionarily enough to allow humans to continue to eat carbohydrates in the massive amounts that everyone, everywhere is eating them.

The Paleo Diet is a recent addition to the low carb diet choice. The ketogenic diet is the ultimate in a low carb diet and has already shown numerous benefits for better health. It's the recommended diet for Celiac Disease since Celiac Disease is caused by the gluten that's found in wheat, barley and rye and a few other grains. It's also the oldest low carb diet, first designed in 1923, to help control seizures. The diet fell out of use when seizure medicines became more prevalent in the 1930s.

It turns out that a ketogenic is the healthiest diet that any human can eat. It goes back to the way our bodies have metabolized food for the last 500,000 years. Simply because this diet is based on fat and not carbs, the diet provides much higher octane fuel for our bodies to use. Carbohydrates have a tendency to gum up your body. They do it by creating plaque and that gets into to the glycation of proteins and LDL cholesterol, which you may remember from *Carbs, How They Cause AGEs* and *Carbs and Arthritis.*

This plaque build-up is the foundation of 75% of the deadliest and costliest diseases, known to man, ranging from breast cancer to Atherosclerosis to 99% of all dementias, making carbohydrates some of the deadliest food that any human can eat. It's not that this food just makes us fat, it kills us slowly and expensively, with an arm long list of disorders. For this one reason alone, the power of being thin cannot be over spoken.

Studies have also shown the simple practice of calorie restriction to have multiple beneficial effects for the body, such as extended life. It's amazing what just going hungry, can do for your body. It not only ramps up your immune system by boosting your anti-oxidants exponentially. While doing that it actually helps your brain grow, with the help of a little protein in your brain known as BDNF, brain derived neurotrophic factor. This is the    protein that makes your brain grow and it doesn't happen as much in obese people. This is part of the power of being thin.

Calorie restriction on a carbohydrate diet is next to impossible, yet I do it every day and quite easily and comfortably, while on my MCT ketogenic diet. An MCT ketogenic diet is, in my estimation, the easiest low carbohydrate diet to get adjusted to. MCTs (Medium Chain Triglycerides) work differently in your body than LCTs (Long Chain Triglycerides). MCTs are a good way to actually lower your cholesterol because they build up the HDL cholesterol. Coconut oil is optimal for this, as it contains lauric acid  and lauric acid is the foundation of HDL cholesterol, the good cholesterol.

Going back to what Dr Miller, had included in his paper, "calorie restriction prolongs life as well as helps to make your brain grow." This is the true power of being thin. It comes easiest from being on a high fat low carb diet.

That means that it's actually healthier to drink whole mile and eat butter again. It's amazing what adding healthy fats back into your diet can do for your overall health. It's nothing short of amazing what it's done for mine. My brain has benefited even more.

Eating cheese is one of the healthiest options you can find, as they're loaded with MCT milk fats. This is the food your body is meant to digest. It's what you were fed  when you were the tiniest baby and it's what you should be eating now. All milk fats are MCT fats and not only give you all the nutrition your body need, but it also helps to keep your weight regulated. (And it doesn't take any effort to stay thin.)

Lactose intolerance quite often is a precursor to diabetes. If you were raised on baby formula, you're addicted to glucose, as it's put in 90% of all baby food. Raw milk is the best milk to drink for people who are lactose intolerant. Because the lactase in the raw milk pre-digests the lactose into fat, your body doesn't have to turn it into fat, as it does with pasteurized milk that doesn't have any lactase.

# Article 21

# WHY NO OUTRAGE? WHY NO WARNING?

When stupid people do stupid things, it has a tendency to catch people's attention. As with the recent acts of terrorism. Stupid people acting as bullies, being stupid. Their tactics only work when we agree to be as stupid as them, and be afraid. That's how bullies work, through fear, and if you don't fear them, their tactics won't work.

We're all outraged about terrorism and the number of lives it's taken and continues to take, which is understandable. Acts of terrorism are usually emotionally senseless acts of violence done simply for political or personal gain. There's absolutely no rationality to it, except for fear. The only goal is to instill fear. This how bullies work....if you allow them.

Why is it, we're so afraid of terrorism? Terrorism in itself might be responsible for almost 0.3% of all deaths. We stand a much more chance of suffering and dying just by getting on the freeway, or easier yet, by simply continuing to eat our comfort foods.

According to Wikipedia "as of 2002, the percentage of deaths, from intentional injuries, i.e. war, violence and suicide was 2.84%". Terrorism as bad as it is, has yet to claim as many lives each year, as either heart disease or cancer or obesity or type 2 diabetes or Alzheimer's disease alone. As bad as terrorism was last year, it still hadn't claimed a million lives. yet cancer alone, was responsible for over 8.2 million deaths or 14.6% of all human deaths in 2012. That's 22,465 deaths per day, worldwide, due to cancer. Heart disease was the number one cause of death with 17.3 million deaths in 2013. That was 47,397 deaths per day. "In 2002 it was responsible for 29.34% of all deaths. In 2013, it was up to 31.5 %."

1/2 of all cancers can be linked to excessive carbohydrate consumption. 1/2 of all cardiovascular diseases can be linked to excessive carbohydrates consumption.

**ECC - Excessive Carbohydrate Consumption is responsible for as much as 42% of all deaths, a minimum of 24 million deaths each year.**

I know that sounds outrageous. I think it is outrageous. Yet, I never hear any outrage, about the number of people's lives that these diseases claim. Allow me to show you exactly how these grain based foods - breads, cereals and pastas (high starch carbs), if removed from the diet, would reduce the occurrence of these diseases by a minimum of 80%. Yes, a reduction of 80% in the occurrences of these diseases, in aggregate, simply by removing the excessive consumption of high starch carbohydrate foods from our diet. Why isn't this treated as a medical condition? It has a very simple cure, don't eat these types of food anymore.

Reducing the occurrence of these diseases would have a couple adverse side effects to our society, reducing the need for the medical community to treat these diseases and eliminating the need for diet companies. I haven't researched how big of an industry the diet and health industry is, but it would definitely have an effect on it, and it might force a lot of people to seek alternative employment.

I tend to wonder if this is why most doctors won't discourage their patients from consuming it? I think mostly, it's just a matter of ignorance, They don't know, or they don't want to know because of their own addiction. (Once you kick the addiction, you can see its influence in those who doubt this concept, the most.) Maybe it's because of their patients addiction to it and their fear of losing their patients to their addiction. This happens when the addiction speaks louder than a patient's personal health, the patient will find a doctor who will treat them with pills or surgery instead of giving up their addiction. That in itself, is proof of the addictive nature of this food.

### 4,100,000 Preventable Deaths From Cancer Each Year!

### Where's the outrage?

When you add cancer deaths of over 8.2 million in 2012, half of which are linked to diet, to the 17,3 million deaths from heart disease, 90% of which are preventable, that adds up to 25.5 million deaths each year, 77% of which are completely preventable. That's 19.67% of all deaths, worldwide, each year are completely preventable and it doesn't count the deaths from any of the other diseases that come from being obese or from having type 2 diabetes or type 3 diabetes, Alzheimer's disease and dementia, which are completely preventable also.

After experiencing what I've experienced and researching what I've researched, I can link 1/2 of all cancers directly to diet. With that said, combine 4.1 million deaths from cancer that could be saved with the 90% of the 17.3 million deaths from heart diseases (15,570,000) and you get a total of 19,670,000 deaths each year that are completely preventable, simply by making a simple yet major diet change. Don't yield to the addiction of this food and buy into the lifetime of need to purchase drugs to combat the diseases that these foods cause.

### 5,000,000 Preventable, Undignified Deaths From Alzheimer's Disease Each Year!

### Where's The Outrage?

It's hard to say exactly how many people die from Alzheimer's disease. With a life expectancy of just six years after diagnosis and with between 21 million and 35 million (as of 2010), having the disease, that means that there will be approximately another 30 million deaths (give or take 3-5 million) from Alzheimer's disease alone, within the next 6 years. That's 5 million each year, 90% of those diseases are preventable. I never hear any outrage about the number of people's lives that these diseases claim.

### 15.570,000 Preventable Deaths From Cardiovascular Disease Each Year!

### Where's the outrage?

According to Wikipedia, "Cardiovascular diseases are the leading cause of death globally. This is true in all areas of the world except Africa. Together they resulted in 17.3 million deaths (31.5%) in 2013 up from 12.3 million (25.8%) in 1990." "It is estimated that 90% of CVD is preventable. Prevention of atherosclerosis is by decreasing risk factors through: healthy eating, exercise, avoidance of tobacco smoke and limiting alcohol intake." 90% of 17.3 is 15.57 which attributes to 15.57 million deaths, due to heart diseases that are preventable. That, to me is nothing short of astounding, yet where's the outrage?

Although relatively few die from obesity alone (usually because the obesity leads to something worse, first), it leads into so many other diseases, that it is indirectly attributable to more deaths than many of these other diseases.

161

Type 2 diabetes, obesity's first disease of death, is what leads into many cancers and heart diseases alone and is why its danger is unparalleled. That's why its control is paramount. If you can control type2 diabetes, you can control every disease it plays a part in. And, it plays a part in most of the deadliest diseases; half dozen cancers, half dozen cardiovascular or heart diseases. And most importantly, it happens in the ones that kill the most people.

Looking at just cancer and cardiovascular disease, they're responsible for more than 25.5 million deaths a year as of 2013. Half of those deaths are due to high carbohydrate consumption, either directly of indirectly. Usually it's indirectly and that is where the trouble lies. Because it is indirectly, it's practically unseen. It was unseen until Dr Davis and Dr Perlmutter uncovered all the evidence. Studies were done and the results (evidence) were quietly stored away for years, with little notice that the studies that produced the evidence ever got published or even announced that they existed.

But there was enough evidence there to influence these doctors to write two books about the danger, *Wheat Belly* and *Grain Brain*. I had already quit eating bread before I read Wheat Belly, but as I read it, it was validating everything that was happening to my body, since I gave it up. *Wheat Belly* led me to *Grain Brain,* which gave me the tools that I needed to piece this book together.

But I must give credit where credit is due. Dr Daniel Amen had persuaded me to give up bread after reading his book *Use Your Brain to Change Your Age*. In his book, he spent more time talking about eating a healthy diet, than any other one thing. At least, that was his lengthiest chapter. It was Thanksgiving 2013 and I weighed 195 lbs at the time, 40lbs more than what I carry now.

After working out extensively for 6 years and not being able to get past the first 30 lbs I lost, in the first month I had started, I decided that it must be my diet. I was eating healthy, very healthy, I thought. It wasn't until I quit eating bread that I found out just how unhealthy it really was. After losing 5 lbs in one month after quitting bread, I decided to give up all grains. When I mention bread, I'm talking about all bread and cereal products, including pasta, crackers and breakfast foods. If it was made of wheat, I wouldn't touch it. In only one month I dropped to a weight, lower than what's prescribed for my height (175 lbs), I was at 165 lbs when I decided to quit all grain foods. I lost another 10 lbs, down to 155lbs. That's about where I "hover" now. I say hover because my weight fluctuates with what I'm doing with my diet. Today, for example, my weight is down to about 151lbs, because I've been on a calorie restriction diet for the last 45 days since I started writing this blog. This action alone has been more beneficial for my brain, in particular, than anything I've ever done for it in my lifetime. Of course it's done wonders for my body and my immune system. When I go hungry I'm creating Ghrelin in my stomach. I can feel the hunger pangs right now, but I'd rather sit here and write, than get up and get something to eat.

I've learned that it's those hunger pangs that tells me my stomach is creating the Ghrelin that activates BDNF in my brain which in turn is building me a bigger and better brain. Everything I've done in the last 45 days has virtually proven what this diet can achieve, something a carbohydrate diet can't. When you read my about me page, and compare that to what I've accomplished in the last 45 days since I started this blog, it's astonishing. At least it is to me. I have never been able to do anything like this before in my entire life. Nobody ever thought I could ever do this after my brain injury 31 years ago. I never thought I could do it. I had always thought, brain cells don't grow back. At least it had made a nice excuse for me, for all the fubars I was responsible for.

That was until I read Dr Perlmutter's book *Grain Brain* and learned that you actually can grow brain cells. I learned that thinner people have bigger brains and that calorie restriction helps build brain cells and new neural networks to connect those cells. It just takes the right formula, a formula that doesn't include any grains or starches.

**High starch food just doesn't have enough nutrition to compensate for the overload of glucose it pours into your system.**

The system it starts with is your digestive system. Then it moves to your circulatory system where it can affect every other system, and then your brain, pancreas and kidneys and eventually most all other organs, until it give us the statistics above. Since the most ubiquitous forms of these diseases involve inflammation, and these foods are the major cause of inflammation (if not only), doesn't it make sense that if you removed these foods from the diet, you would remove a major cause of the diseases that are influenced by it?

**Why are they still promoted like they are?**

**Where's the recommendation**

**from more doctors to stop eating it?**

**There's absolutely no rationality to it, except addiction.**

# Where's the outrage?

To see how removing carbs out of the diet of everyone worldwide could lead to the end of terrorism worldwide, read article 26 *My Thoughts on the Eradication of Carbs From Our Society.*

# PART III


# SOCIETAL CONCERNS

# ARTICLE 22

# INDUSTRY'S CONCERN ABOUT THE DISPELLING OF WHEAT AND GRAINS

What moves America forward, more than anything else, is corporate advancement. Hence the control of corporations in the America, is what drives this advancement.

If any major change is to occur within the realms of modern society, it must be done, on a corporate level. This brings us to the dilemma of how to change the behavior of millions of people, all who are addicted to these substances and worse yet addicted to what corporate America tells them. Corporate America tells them what to think as well as how to think. It tells them what to wear, how to eat, what to drink. By strategically placing their influence in food and drink, this puts them in control of the amount of sugar we consume, which in turn, controls our emotions, to put us 'under their spell', so to speak. They're never going to want to give that up. That's something that we have to take back. and that's why I registered the url for the website this book came from, www.saveourdignity.org.

In order to effect, changes in the food industry, primarily the grain industry, we need to make the food industrial complex of America understand, that we're tired of this abuse. It must be incorporated into this network of our society, that change must happen. The problem therein lies, the size of this industry is huge. It's comprised of, probably more companies, than any other industry, in the world, as food is the most important commodity that's marketed worldwide. The number of companies within this industry is almost unimaginable. So how do we change the behavior of this much of our society? It can't be done overnight. It's going to take the efforts of everyone in society, to make a change, this grandiose, which means it's going to take a while.

Corporate industry, the food industry primarily, must confront the dangers, that they are imposing on the entire world, by continuing to grow, manufacture, market, advertise and sell this devastating food that causes so many illnesses and diseases. They must understand that killing their customers, is not a solid business plan.

I realize that many of the crop seed companies, (Monsanto, Dupont Pioneer, Syngenta, Land O' Lakes, Bayer and many other overseas), had a lot of the money tied up in pharmaceuticals, as well as manufacturing the crop seed, (much of it genetically modified). Even though many of those companies liquidated their investments in the pharmaceutical side of the industry, many of these companies still have ties to each other, which begs the question, were cover-ups instigated to help hide these facts? It conjures, in my mind, the question of how threatened did they feel if any of this information was released to the public? Are these valid arguments? I think so. And I think, they deserve further investigation. This endeavor, is where it gets interesting. With corporate America in so much control of how our society functions, it's occurred to me that nothing is going to happen, until corporate America, the food industry and pharmaceutical industry, in general change their behavior, They must discontinue the marketing and advertising of these products, so as to not persuade the public that they need to continue to eat this garbage. The question arises, how do you make a company cut its own throat. Because if anything were to interrupt the flow of their finances, how long can they stay in business? This brings us to the core of what we need to work toward to change, and changing it, may result in much of this industry disappearing.

The drink industry, for example, they're probably the most guilty of any, for slipping this dangerous food into our diet, by loading up their drinks with *high fructose corn syrup, sugar, Aspartame, Cyclamate, Saccharin, Sucralose, Acesulfame potassium, malt syrup, Lead acetate, and many other that I have trouble pronouncing, like maltodextrin, maltitol, maltotriose, Icodextrin,* and too many forms of oligosaccharides to list here. To find them all, you need to refer to every food label on every can of soft drink, that's on the market. Convincing the beverage industry of finding other sources of sweeteners is already beginning to take place. A lot of manufacturers are starting to offer drinks sweetened with Stevia, a completely natural, non-caloric sweetener, that's concentrated, when it's offered in powdered form. My wish, is for the transformation of all sweetened drinks to Stevia instead of the high sugar sweeteners, like all of those listed above. Can you imagine what this would do, to get this dangerous substance out of our diet?    I can.

So how do we replace the lost business and everything else that goes along with it, the jobs and careers, the investment of millions of Americans, who've all invested in these companies(through their *IRA's,* Keoghs, investment funds, etc). How do we take away all of that? The problem is, you can't, and that's where the problem of dispelling this problem lies. You have to replace what you take away, with healthier options, healthier for the body, healthier for the mind, healthier for business and corporate America. My contention is that America, and the health of the individual run hand in hand. They depend on each other. They're crucial to each other's survival.

Why then, doesn't the food industry understand this basic fundamental law of business, that killing your customers with inferior products, is killing your industry? Unless that industry is still working with the pharmaceutical industry, like they were 20 years ago. Could they be that indebted to the pharmaceutical industry, that they have to keep sending them customers? Man O man does this open up a can of worms, making the construction of that article, an endeavor that I can't wish upon anyone! But, I'm going to try to untangle this quagmire, so stay tuned. The eradication of this dangerous carbohydrate out of our diet, is going to take a global effort, because of its presence, everywhere. But with the help of industry, it might be possible to just do so.

# ARTICLE 23

# INDUSTRY'S INFLUENCE IN THE EXPANSION OF CARB PRODUCTION

It would be nice if money weren't the primary motivating factor in business. It would be nice of the health and welfare of every individual human being were the primary motivating factor in business. But it's not. That is why this article may be the hardest one to construct. It not only involves corporate America, it involves a major portion of all industry. both big and small, Even down to the mom and pop stores in small town, America, and that's what makes this post so hard to write.

The problem is, it invades the very core of our society, our sustenance. This is what we all work for. Our primary goal, for our families, (after finding shelter) is to put food on the table. And this is where the problem begins. Everyone has to eat. This makes everyone, who's hungry, susceptible to outside influences, to quench those hunger pangs.

The food industry understands this. They've done numerous studies on it. Their research has told them how, when, where, and to whom to market their products to. All so they can increase their profits.

Their only interest, though, is to please their stockholders, they're not interested in their customers health (except for a few in the health industry), so everything they do, is done for the bottom line, profit. Because of this shortsightedness, and not looking that far into the future, they're cutting their own throats, by crippling their buyers with products, that are not only making their customers sick, their products are killing the customers. (Not a good business plan)

These products kill because of the sugar they contain, we all know that. But the problem here is that they don't kill immediately, so they're legal. Their death sentence takes a lot longer. It's a lot more painful. It's a lot more expensive. It's a lot more emotionally draining. Many times it's more violent. It's definitely, nothing anyone should have to experience, yet the addiction, keeps anyone who's on this diet, remain on this diet, voluntarily. Only those strong enough, can break the cycle of addiction. But the beauty of breaking it, is this, it doesn't take that long, as long as you can abstain from its lure. It only takes a month or two, for the average addict. Heavier, more addicted people, might take another month or two.

Bringing the food industry to an understanding, that they are sacrificing tomorrows customers for today's profits, may help in curbing corporate influence , but is it enough to change the behavior of all corporate America? I don't know. The amount of change that would have to occur, is enormous, because the industry which is enormous. How do you change an industry this enormous? The only way I know how to, is one company at a time, until all companies see the light.

Unfortunately, profit doesn't have a soul. It has no moral values. And it's the moral values that make us a society. Without them, we'd have no laws or regulations to keep people from stepping on other people's toes. This begs the question, what role does profit play in a civilized culture. Most of us know that profit = money. Most of us also know that a civilization needs money to conduct commerce, so everyone within that civilization can trade their goods and services. It's this trade, that's at the core of civilization. People came together in primitive times for protection, and this, in turn, started us trading our possessions and food. And thus, the beginning of commerce, the engine that keeps our society, culture and civilization growing.

If, it's the desire of money, that's at the root of all evil, does that make all of corporate America evil, because of their desire to improve their profits? Some would say so, simply because of the lack of responsibility corporate America takes for their actions when they harm others. Others would say, it's survival. In all actuality, it's both. The desire for profit and power, is what drives almost all of corporate America. It's my opinion, that this is where corporate America is failing society.

Because they have to fulfill stockholders wishes to make more money, they are obligated to do so. Doing anything else would not be considered profitable and it wouldn't keep the stockholders happy. The company would lose the investment of their stockholders and this in turn would strongly disable their ability to conduct business and therein threaten the existence of the company. Profit is important. It's one of the biggest, if not the biggest motivating factors in our society.

We, in the United States, have always used our freedoms, to bolster our efforts to increase our profits. It's this freedom, that's built the strongest empire in history. The problem is this, when you consider freedom and what it brings us, you have to look at the other side of the coin, that freedom is on. The other side of this freedom coin, that's tossed around so much (mostly politically), is responsibility. You can't have true freedom without responsibility. The responsibility side of the coin, says, that you must take responsibility for the freedoms you enjoy, especially when those freedoms inflict harm on another human being. You can't have true freedom without this responsibility.

Without the responsibility, what do you have? A society without control. When any one person, group, or company isn't fully responsible for enjoying their freedoms, where does the freedom exist, for all parties? In that sense then, where does it exist for anyone? It doesn't, when one does harm to any other person or group. This is where the problem lies. Only one person's freedom was expressed. The person on whom this expression of freedom was committed, wasn't allowed to express their own freedom, because they were subjected to the freedoms of the other. Is this really true freedom? I submit, that it isn't, it's not true freedom at all. At best, it's pseudo freedom and it sounds a lot like slavery.

It's how our system, works, and because our Supreme Court thinks that corporations are the same as people, they deserve the same rights and freedoms as any single individual human being. Do corporations have the same morals as most human beings? Yet, their allowed a lot more freedom, simply because, they have the money to do so.

Here's the worst part of this, equation. It's because of your addiction. It's your money they use. You give it to them, freely, every time you buy their products. At least you think you do. What you think is your own choice, to purchase what you think is healthy food, is actually you succumbing to their desire. You are slaves to their wishes, every time you bag their groceries…and later on years down the road, their drugs.

This is a trap, that I refuse to fall into. I can only thank Dr Perlmutter, Dr Davis, and Dr Amen, for setting me on the path that brought me to this point, and this book, (I don't mention Dr Amen anywhere in any of my articles, except right here. The reason I mention him here, is because, he's the one who basically started me on this journey.)

Carbohydrates are a food of emotion. It's how they make you fat. They control your emotions. They'll continue to control your emotions until you give them up and in thus doing control them. There's a certain corporation with the intention of owning all farming industry in America and in doing so has tainted you carbs far beyond recognition, but you have to read *A Cure for the World* to understand how they're doing that. Total control of our food supply to control what you eat. I only let GOD control me. Who do you let control you?

171

# ARTICLE 24

# THE EFFECTS OF CARBOHYDRATES ON OUR SOCIETY THROUGHOUT HISTORY AND TODAY

We owe our civilization to the dawn of agriculture. It was the beginning of agriculture, which started civilization because it transformed our ancestors into a people who didn't need to move around to find food. They didn't have to. They learned how to grow it. And this is where the problem of today, started. It started at the same time civilization, as a whole, started over 10,000 years ago. That's the reason it's woven, so tightly into our society. As important as it's been to our society, in the past, it's that important to curb our use of it in our diet, now. As well as it has served us in the past as a food source, we need to curb its use now, because of the damage this new modern food is doing to our health and emotions.

Never in our entire history, has this food that we've been eating for over 10,000 years, been as dangerous as it is today. Don't misunderstand me it's always been dangerous, in the respect that it creates such massive changes in the sugar levels of most mammals. And because of that, it creates the glucose that creates the fat that creates the glycation that creates the plaque that creates the CVDs and cancers. It's the way our biology works and there's no getting around it.

The food source that I'm referring to here is wheat. It was one of the founding crops that we grew, and it's helped develop our civilizations, throughout history. It's also helped to destroy civilizations throughout history by keeping us hungry. And the way it did it, was due to the same quality of this food that makes it so dangerous today. That's its ability to fluctuate sugar levels in all who ingest it. That's why cattle ranchers use grains, to fatten their herds. Grains, in general, are fattening foods. It was important in ancient times to eat fattening foods. We needed the fat to tide us over in times when food was scarce. Now, food isn't scarce. It's not even hard to get. As a matter of fact, this kind of food has become far too easy to get and that's where the danger lies. This food is far too available. Food like this was never this available in the quantities we eat them, for our ancestors. They had to work to either find their food, or grow their food. It just didn't come to them as easy as we are able to get our hands on it. Because of this, the bodies that used to have to exercise to get their food don't have to today. But that only presents one reason, that what sustained us throughout history is killing us today, out of many. There're actually multiple reasons.

This #1 reason, that's been with us since wheat's inception, is the fact that it's a carbohydrate. The other reason, you can blame on genetic engineering. Genetic modifying has made it a product, now, that's high in starchy non-nutritious carbs with very limited added nutrient content. What nutrients it has are not worth the trade-off of the massive amounts of carbohydrates you get when you eat this food. But the fact that it's a carbohydrate in the first place, is at the root of the problem. The problem is that carbohydrates are metabolized on a cellular level, with the hormone insulin. This turns the carbohydrate into fat so it can enter the cell, to be used as a fuel. It's here, that the

173

problem begins. The fat, that the insulin turns the carbohydrate into, is not that good of a fat. It is fat your body would rather store than use right away. This primitive digestive behavior is coupling itself with today's sedentary lifestyles, to produce disastrous results.

Those results are what are costing you millions of lives, dollars, hours in lost production, as well as complete losses of your mental and emotional senses. All this is due to the way this food controls our blood sugars. When eaten by humans, they're subject to the fluctuations of their blood glucose, due to the glucose infusion in the blood stream, setting off the cry for insulin. But we're not going to talk about insulin, because it's part of the story doesn't come back in, until you start looking what this food has the ability to do to you. This is the reason for all the illness and diseases it's causing today. If you doubt this, by now, you're listening to your hormones and letting them control your emotions. I can understand, I was there just a few years ago.

What we're going to look at is the change in blood glucose in the body and what influences it has on one's emotions, thoughts, actions and speech as well as physical and mental health. We're going to do this because the food we've been ingesting throughout our entire lifetime, as a species, is supposed to be the same food we're eating right now, when in all actuality, it's not. The food we're eating now, that resembles this staple of our diet for so many years, isn't anything like that of what we ate then. Today's version of this staple is much higher in fat causing carbohydrates, than what it used to be in the past. It's this one little factor about its existence that sets it aside from all other foods. The simple fact, because it has the ability to change your blood glucose, it has the ability to change your emotional patterns, as well as behavioral patterns. Who knows what influence this factor has had throughout history? I can see today, how those patterns have been amplified. They've been amplified, because the food that causes this behavior has been amplified in the amount of carbohydrates it provides, to those who eat it. Their glucose levels are always varying by wide margins which in turn makes their emotions vary by wide margins also. This variance in range of emotions, is what I contend, is a major influence in worldwide behavior today.

I wonder what it would be like if everyone were on a keto diet and weren't subject to the glucose changes in the blood and thereby not subject to changes in their emotional behavior. Would everyone think and behave more rationally? I contend that they would. I know I have since I've been on a keto diet. It's done so much to alter my emotional behavior that it's made me a completely new person. I'm not nearly as volatile as I used to be. I don't lose my temper like I used to. Most importantly, I don't get frustrated as much as I used to. Simply put, I'm a much saner guy, than what I used to be. I think much more rationally, now that I'm on a keto diet. If this diet can do this for me, can you imagine what it can do for anyone else? I try to imagine what it could do for the world and how it might help to mellow everyone out, just a little bit. It would, at least, make everyone healthier and that change alone, might go a long way to evening our emotions. Most importantly, it will cut hunger, which goes a long way to controlling emotions.

**My contention is that it can do it for me, it can do it for anybody in the world and if it can, why can't that change the behavior of the world?**

Only abstinence from this food, can tell us if it would work. I ask you, why not try it? See find out if I'm correct in my assumptions? What do we have to lose? Bad Health? Lost production? Lost wealth? Lost sanity? Lost dignity? To me the trade off is worth the gamble, wouldn't you think so?

I've learned that the human body has a miraculous ability to heal and cure itself, if you give it a chance. I've also learned, that chance can't include carbs. For me, and you it's either the cure, or the carbs, not both. It's your choice.

## THE TIME HAS COME FOR A CURE

## THE CURE BEGINS WITH YOUR CHOICES

# ARTICLE 25

# CARBS. THE ARGUMENT FOR THEM

How many of you would be afraid to tell your doctor, that you would like to go on a high fat, low carb diet? How many of you are afraid, yourself, to go on a Paleo or ketogenic diet? If I had to make a guess, as to how many of you answered "I am" to this question, I would wager it's probably above 90% and I can't say that I blame you. The information contained within this book and my website and all the others, that expound the virtues of the ketogenic diet, and the pitfalls of a carbohydrate diet are, in the least, alarming, at the mean, it's staggering. but at the most, it's nothing short of amazing or even deadly. And that's why I'm writing this book. I honestly think it's time that we look at the root reason for the problems that exist in society, today, sugar and carbohydrates.

I apologize. I didn't want to start this page with a paragraph like that. I would have much rather started it out with all the benefits that carbohydrates provide.

**Problem is, there's only 1.**

A small part of your brain needs glucose to function. It can't operate on ketones. When your brain needs this glucose, though, it can get it from your liver and muscles. This is called **gluconeogenesis**. This is where your body manufacturers glucose for your brain, from muscle and .liver tissue. I've read accounts where the author expressed fear of muscle tissue wasting away under these conditions. This is the furthest from the truth, of what actually happens.

The question I ask myself is, how can my muscle waste away, if I'm supplying it with enough protein to replace whatever my brain takes? Being on a diet high in protein, is going to keep any muscle tissue wasting away from gluconeogenesis. This is a process my body is truly blessed to have, an unending source of what little glucose my brain needs. I can now rest with the comfort of knowing that I don't ever have to put this poison in my body again.

According to Dr, Perlmutter, on page 23 of his best seller, *Grain Brain,* "the body can manufacture glucose from fat or protein, if necessary through a process called gluconeogenesis". Dr. Perlmutter also has stated in one of his you tube videos, that he believes that the human body can live without any carbohydrate infusion at all.

For the last two years, last 6 months in particular, I've reduced the glucose level in my blood to levels which, in turn, have reduced the inflammation and pain in my body far under the levels it was prior, it's kept my weight 15 to 20 pounds below my recommended weight, given me more energy, kept my emotions level, dropped my need for medication to zilch, and although I hinted at this before, allowed me to sit at my desk and work for 16 to 20 hours a day for the last four days, while only taking short brakes to nibble a few snacks. I've had no meals in the past four days. I had a total of 12 hour of sleep over the last three nights. The point I'm trying to make is that, being on a ketogenic diet will allow the body to go through the stress that I've been putting mine through. This is something that can't be done, on a diet high in carbohydrates. This is something that can't be done on a carbohydrate diet at all, especially if those carbohydrates include grains. It's that simple, carbs kill because sugar kills. And they're best at killing energy. All this is due to their addictive nature.

# BREAK THE ADDICTION TO

# FREE YOURSELF FROM BEING THEIR SLAVE.

# ARTICLE 26

# WHY NO OUTRAGE? WHY NO WARNING?

When stupid people do stupid things, it has a tendency to catch people's attention. As with the recent acts of terrorism. Stupid people acting as bullies, being stupid. Their tactics only work when we agree to be as stupid as them, and be afraid. That's how bullies work, through fear, and if you don't fear them, their tactics won't work.

We're all outraged about terrorism and the number of lives it's taken and continues to take, which is understandable. Acts of terrorism are quite often angry acts of violence done simply for political or personal gain. There's absolutely no rationality to it, except for fear. The only goal is to instill fear. This is how bullies work….if you allow them.

Why is it, we're so afraid of terrorism? Terrorism in itself might
be responsible for almost 0.3% of all deaths. We stand a much more chance
of suffering and dying just by getting on the freeway, or easier yet, by simply
continuing to eat our comfort foods.

According to Wikipedia *"as of 2002, the percentage of death from intentional injuries, i.e. war, violence and suicide  was 2.84%"*.  Terrorism as bad as it is, has yet to claim as many lives each year, as either heart disease or cancer or obesity or type 2 diabetes or Alzheimer's disease, alone! As bad as terrorism was last year, it still hadn't claimed a million lives. yet cancer alone, was responsible for over 8.2 million deaths or 14.6% of all human deaths in 2012. That's 22,465 deaths per day, worldwide, due to cancer. Heart disease was the number one cause of death with 17.3 million deaths in 2013. That was 47,397 deaths per day. *"In 2002 it was responsible for 29.34% of all deaths."*  In 2013, it was up to 31.5 %.

1/2 of all cancers can be linked to excessive carbohydrate consumption. 1/2 of all cardiovascular diseases can be linked to excessive carbohydrate consumption.

**ECC - Excessive Carbohydrate Consumption is responsible for as much as 42% of all deaths, a minimum of 24 million deaths each year.**

Roy Knight Jr

I know that sounds outrageous. I think it is outrageous. Yet, I never hear any outrage, about the number of people's lives that these diseases claim. Allow me to show you exactly how these grain based foods - breads, cereals and pastas (high starch carbs), sugary drinks, and alcohol, were removed from the diet, would reduce the occurrence of these diseases by a minimum of 80%. Yes, a reduction of 80% in the occurrences of these diseases, in aggregate, simply by removing the excessive consumption of high starch carbohydrate foods, sugary drinks and alcohol, from our diet. Why isn't this treated as a medical condition? It has a very simple cure, don't eat these types of food anymore.

Reducing the occurrence of these diseases would have a couple adverse side effects to our society, reducing the need for the medical community to treat these diseases and eliminating the need for diet companies. I haven't researched how big of an industry the diet and health industry is, but it would definitely have an effect on it, and it might force a lot of people to seek alternative employment....but that would probably take a few centuries.

I tend to wonder if this is why most doctors won't discourage their patients from consuming it? I think mostly, it's just a matter of ignorance, They don't know, or they don't want to know because of their own addiction. (Once you kick the addiction, you can see its influence in those who doubt this concept, the most.) Maybe it's because of their patients addiction to it and their fear of losing their patients to their addiction. This happens when the addiction speaks louder than a patient's personal health, the patient will find a doctor who will treat them with pills or surgery instead of giving up their addiction. That in itself, is proof of the addictive nature of this food.

**4,100,000 Preventable Deaths From Cancer Each Year!**

**Where's the outrage?**

When you add cancer deaths of over 8.2 million in 2012, half of which are linked to diet, to the 17,3 million deaths from heart disease, 90% of which are preventable, that adds up to 25.5 million deaths each year, 77% of which are completely preventable. That's 19.67% of all deaths, worldwide, each year are completely preventable and that doesn't count the deaths from any of the other diseases that come from being obese or from having type 2 diabetes or type 3 diabetes, Alzheimer's disease and dementia, which are completely preventable also.

## 5,000,000 Preventable, Undignified Deaths From Alzheimer's Disease Each Year!

### Where's The Outrage?

It's hard to say exactly how many people die from Alzheimer's disease. With a life expectancy of just six years after diagnosis and with between 21 million and 35 million (as of 2010), having the disease, that means that there will be approximately another 30 million deaths (give or take 3-5 million) from Alzheimer's disease alone, within the next 6 years. That's 5 million each year, 90% of those diseases are preventable. I never hear any outrage about the number of people's lives that these diseases claim.

After experiencing what I've experienced and researching what I've researched, I can link 1/2 of all cancers directly to diet. With that said, combine 4.1 million deaths from cancer that could be saved with the 90% of the 17.3 million deaths from heart diseases (15,570,000) and you get a total of 19,670,000 deaths each year that are completely preventable, simply by making a simple yet major diet change. Don't yield to the addiction of this food and buy into the lifetime of need to purchase drugs to combat the diseases that these foods cause.

### 15,570,000 Preventable Deaths From Cardiovascular Disease Each Year!        Where's the outrage?

According to Wikipedia, *"Cardiovascular diseases are the leading cause of death globally. This is true in all areas of the world except Africa. Together they resulted in 17.3 million deaths (31.5%) in 2013 up from 12.3 million (25.8%) in 1990." "It is estimated that 90% of CVD is preventable. Prevention of atherosclerosis is by decreasing risk factors through: healthy eating, exercise, avoidance of tobacco smoke and limiting alcohol intake."* 90% of 17.3 is 15.57 which attributes to 15.57 million deaths, due to heart diseases that are preventable. That, to me is nothing short of astounding, yet where's the outrage?

Although relatively few die from obesity alone (usually because the obesity leads to something worse, first), it leads into so many other diseases, that it is indirectly attributable to more deaths than many of these other diseases. Type 2 diabetes, obesity's first disease of death, is what leads into many cancers and heart diseases alone and is why its danger is unparalleled.

That's why its control is paramount. If you can control type2 diabetes, you can control every disease it plays a part in. And, it plays a part in most of the deadliest diseases; half dozen cancers, half dozen cardiovascular or heart diseases. And most importantly, it happens in the ones that kill the most people.

Looking at just cancer and cardiovascular disease, they're responsible for more than 25.5 million deaths a year as of 2013. Half of those deaths are due to high carbohydrate consumption, either directly of indirectly. Usually it's indirectly and that is where the trouble lies. Because it is indirectly, it's practically unseen. It was unseen until Dr Davis and Dr Perlmutter uncovered all the evidence. Studies were done and the results (evidence) were quietly stored away for years, with little notice that the studies that produced the evidence ever got published or even announced that they existed.

But there was enough evidence there to influence these doctors to write two books about the danger, *Wheat Belly* and *Grain Brain.* I had already quit eating bread before I read Wheat Belly, but as I read it, it was validating everything that was happening to my body, since I gave it up. *Wheat Belly* led me to *Grain Brain,* which gave me the tools that I needed to piece this book together.

But I must give credit where credit is due. Dr Daniel Amen had persuaded me to give up bread after reading his book *Use Your Brain to Change Your Age.* In his book, he spent more time talking about eating a healthy diet, than any other one thing. At least, that was his lengthiest chapter. It was Thanksgiving 2013 and I weighed 195 lbs at the time, 40+lbs more than what I carry now.

After working out extensively for 6 years and not being able to get past the first 30 lbs I lost, in the first month I had started, I decided that it must be my diet. I was eating healthy, very healthy, I thought. It wasn't until I quit eating bread that I found out just how **unhealthy** it really was. After losing 5 lbs in one month after quitting bread, I decided to give up all grains. When I mention bread, I'm talking about all bread and cereal products, including pasta, crackers and breakfast foods. If it was made of wheat, I wouldn't touch it.

In only another  month I dropped to a weight, lower than what's prescribed for my height (175 lbs), I was at 165 lbs when I decided to quit all grain foods. I lost another 10 lbs, down to 155lbs. That's about where I "hover" now. I say hover because my weight fluctuates with what I'm doing with my diet. Today, for example, my weight is down to about 151lbs, because I've been on a calorie restriction diet for the last 45 days since I started writing this book. This action alone has been more beneficial for my brain, in particular, than anything I've ever done for it in my lifetime. Of course it's done wonders for my body and my immune system. When I go hungry I'm creating Ghrelin in my stomach. I can feel the hunger pangs right now, but I'd rather sit here and write, than get up and get something to eat.

I've learned that it's those hunger pangs that tells me my stomach is creating the Ghrelin that activates *BDNF* in my brain which in turn is building me a bigger and better brain. Everything I've done in the last 45 days has virtually proven what this diet can achieve, something a carbohydrate diet can't. When you read my about me page, and compare that to what I've accomplished in the last 45 days since I published my website, it's astonishing. At least it is to me. I have never been able to do anything like this before in my entire life. Nobody ever thought I could ever do this after my brain injury 31 years ago. I never thought I could do it. I had always thought, brain cells don't grow back. At least it had made a nice excuse for me, for all the fubars I was responsible for.

That was until I read Dr Perlmutter's book *Grain Brain* and learned that you actually can grow brain cells. I learned that thinner people have bigger brains and that calorie restriction helps build brain cells and new neural networks to connect those cells. It just takes the right formula, a formula that doesn't include any grains or starches or worse yet, any sugary drinks or alcohol.

**High starch food, sodas, and alcohol just doesn't have enough nutrition to compensate for the overload of glucose it pours into your system.**

The system it starts with is your digestive system. Then it moves to your circulatory system where it can affect every other system, and then your brain, pancreas and kidneys and eventually most all other organs, until it give us all of the statistics above. Since the most ubiquitous forms of these diseases involve inflammation, and these foods are a major (if not only) cause of inflammation, doesn't it make sense that if you removed these foods out of our diet, you would remove a major cause of the diseases that are influenced by it.

183

# ARTICLE 27

## My Thoughts On The Eradication Of Carbs

This is my favorite article. Every time I dream of a world without carbs, I get to add it to this article. There are so many thoughts running through my head, that it's hard to find a place to start this page on how I feel about getting rid of the carbohydrate diet, that not only addicts everyone to this abhorrent behavior, but causes so much damage to our bodies, teeth, emotions, lives, relationships both personal and globally, finances, and mostly importantly, politics, that it makes it very hard to pick a spot to start, so I guess that's what I must do. Let's go back the damage it causes to our bodies, teeth, emotions, lives, relationships, and finances.

I said it often in my first article, *Carbs, The New Death Sentence*, the removal of carbs from the diet and the transition to a diet, higher in fats and proteins, will not only heal a major portion of our population, from most of the inflictions that currently bother them, it will keep everyone healthier and more even tempered, well into the future, simply because of the lack of sugar in the blood. It's that simple. This idea of a society that's not addicted to sugar, is compelling me to dream of the possibilities. I think I need to start a what if, list. What if:

- Nobody in the world ate carbs and suffered from the massive sugar fluctuations in the blood stream, would there be as much violence as there is, in the world today?
- Everybody in the world quit subjecting their emotions to these fluctuations in blood sugar changes, that come with the ingestion of wheat and grain foods, would differences get worked out in a more reasonable way?
- Everyone broke their addiction to this substance and quit eating it, would the grain industry (no pun intended) grind to a halt?
- It never showed up in our diet in the first place, would we have the problems we have today? Or would we be further advanced, and more prepared to find other living arrangements for our expanding population, on another planet in a galaxy, far far away, (when the "apocalypse" comes, that was supposed to happen in 2012)?
- The studies that I've encountered in my research, were ever revealed to the public, after their completion, would we still be experiencing all of the problems that we live with today? Problems of crime, terrorism, abhorrent behavior of any nature? If everyone's blood sugar levels, never

went out of whack, Would any of the violent nature that you see in people today, ever exist?

- It ever got published in any of the popular journals that circulate throughout the medical community, after the research was completed on any of the studies within any of the research I've been fortunate to have been made aware of, by Dr's Davis and Perlmutter, would our medical industry be fashioned in a different manner, so as they wouldn't have to contend with the amount of illness and disease that this food manifests?
- I was introduced to a diet high in fats and proteins when I was young, how many of the ailments would I not be suffering from, now? How deformed would I not be, or would I be, at all?
- Society in whole ate a diet high in protein and fats, would our world have to live through so much turmoil?
- The whole world has been on a keto diet since the beginning of civilization, instead of converting over to a diet of carbohydrates, because agriculture was introduced to our race, when we were primitive, would have all acts of war, conquests, crusades, rebellions, uprisings, riots, violent crime, violent behavior, and worst of all, terrorism ever taken place?
- Due to the lack of outside influence (glucose changes in the blood) influencing behavior and emotional reactions, caused by those fluctuations in the blood sugars, would as much of the violence ever have taken place? I'm willing to wager that a majority of them it not have, simply because the need for them to take place would have never existed. If our race could have grown on a ketogenic diet, would our culture would be as advanced as it is, now? Since it was agriculture that civilized our race, it was agriculture that started our advancement to what we are today. The question I ask now, has our advancement been in any way been restricted because of our addiction to a carbohydrate diet? My guess is, yes. It has. It is. And, it will continue to be, until we kill this addiction.
- The benefit of the whole world being on this diet that doesn't affect emotional behavior so much, would allow emotions to remain much more in tack, making the need for war of terrorism much less necessary?
- The world has the benefit of being on a high protein and fat diet, as opposed to a high carbohydrate diet, since time immemorial, would it have allowed our culture to develop differently because it would have never had to deal with the amount of illness and disease they cause?
- If the world were on a keto diet, Would I have ever suffered from a severe closed head injury, in the first place? Would the drunk, who ran the red light, that hit the car I was riding in, not have been drunk? Would he have

not needed to drink alcohol, because of the better stabilization of his emotions, because he would have been, on a keto diet?

- If the world were on a keto diet, and knew about the sugar problems that alcohol, gives you, would there be the problem that we have with alcohol, today? Or would everyone be better able to resist the temptations, alcohol, brings?

- If the world were on a keto diet, and everyone thought with a clearer head, and were more able to keep their emotions intact, would the amount of disagreements that happen, be settled in more reasonable ways, everywhere? If that were to happen, what would happen to all the violence in the world?

- You could track where a majority of violence occurs, would there be a higher volume of sugar in the diet, there? If sugar can affect our emotions so much, If it were removed from the diet in all areas, that experience violence, would the violence still exist?

- If the world were on a keto diet, what would the medical industry do?

- If the world were on a keto diet, what would the dental industry do?

- If the world were on a keto diet, what would happen to the pharmaceutical industry, grain industry, farming industry

- If the world were on a keto diet, what would happen to the crime rate? Crime is driven by greed and hunger, what would happen if greed and hunger no longer existed, because there are no more changes in our emotional status, caused by the fluctuations in our blood sugars, which are no longer present in the body? What if hunger no longer existed because of our abilities to go longer periods of time between meals, due the states of ketosis our bodies would be in.

- If the world were on a keto diet, what would happen to the terrorism in the world? Most terrorism is caused by the need to retaliate, in any violent form or manner. Since there would be no sugar in the blood to influence behavior, we would be more enabled to control our **emotional behavior**, to the point, that we would be able to settle our differences more peaceably and amicably. This in turn, would go far to eliminate the need for retaliation, which in turn would go a long way to stopping terrorism. It's that simple, remove the carbs, remove the emotional disorder, remove the terrorism. It's that simple. Remove the carbs, remove the violence. (Thank you, Dr Perlmutter!)

Keep in mind, these are only thoughts, questions I keep asking myself. Questions that keep haunting me. So it's my concern, to deal with right now, not yours. Your concern, my only hope is, that you will learn and take heed.

**IT'S TIME TO CURE**

**AMERICA'S WORST ADDICTION**

**GLUCOSE - SUGAR AND CARBS**

**JUST SAY NO TO GLUCOSE**

# FINAL THOUGHTS

I'm sure your asking, why did I include this last article, *Why No Outrage,* 3 times in this book. Thank you for asking that question I appreciate it very much. The answer to that question is the entire reason for writing this book.

I wanted to not only point out how bad these foods are for our physical bodies, I wanted to point out, what that damage of our physiology, has done to our society (of which I have much more to write about), and I wanted to give an idea of the costs to our society. I also wanted to let people know just who is perpetuating this myth, that you need to eat more carbs, so everyone who cares about their health, wealth and most importantly, their dignity, can make wise decisions about how they feed their bodies.

To me, it's all for the almighty buck, which is nothing more than greed....greed for money, greed for power. Corporations have to keep their stockholders happy, and in doing so, have created masterful advertising campaigns telling us just how healthy the food they offer, is, when in all actuality, it isn't, and they know it.

But they're "too big to fail" so they're allowed to lie to the consumer about the qualities of their food products, which are at the least, addictive, at the mean, brain damaging, and at the most, deadly. To me, it's all for the almighty buck, which is nothing more than greed....greed for money, greed for power.

My hope is that you now realize that every piece of bread or sugar you're putting in your body, is filling it with glue to muck it up and keep it from running efficiently. And every time you do that, you bow to their control.

My goal is to impress upon as many people as I can, that our behavior as a society, needs to change. And it needs to change sooner, rather than later, simply for the sake of our society as a whole as well as our climate (farming) and ability to move into the future, productively, instead of destructively.

## So why does it still continue?

## Addiction!

# AFTERTHOUGHTS

I'd like to think, I'm a nobody. Or at least, I used to be. Prior to this book, I've accomplished little, especially in the last 30+ years. I chose to follow a (no carb) ketogenic diet about six months ago. Four months ago I published the basis of this book on a website by the same name. In four days I've reformatted my website, www.saveourdignity.org into this book. I've spent the last 3 weeks editing and proofing my book. That may not sound like much to most of you, but after you read my "about me page" you should have an idea of what I have to live and work with.

I figured this out and I don't have a degree more than an A.A. degree and a digital electronics diploma. Yet, because of my disability, I was motivated enough to try to learn how I could retrieve that which I had lost over 30 years ago to a drunk driver running a red light.

I started writing this book for my mother when I published my website, Curb Your Carbs, and continued writing post after post after post of what I found to be devastating news that I thought the whole world should know.

I used to have learning disabilities that were completely unrecognized 40-50 years ago, when I was young. I was just labeled as a rambunctious typical boy. I walked home from school the first day of my second year. I missed the part where the teacher said she was going to review what we learned the previous year. So at first recess, I walked home, only to have my mother march my right back.

My reason, which I thought valid, was that I wasn't learning anything new. It was the same stuff that we learned last year and I thought, I've got better things to do than to sit here and relearn what I already know, so I walked home, where I had better things to do.

I didn't realize this, at the time. Neither did my mother. But it was a sign of my ADD. This ADD that I was inflicted with, I can see now was a direct result of my diet, which happened to be a diet high in carbohydrates.

Actually, it was very high in carbs. Mom thought, that's what she was supposed to feed us. It's what she fed her siblings when she had to take care of them, after her father died, when she was 12 and her mother had to go to work to support the family.

At that time, this food that she unwittingly addicted us to was not nearly as dangerous as it is today. Today it's been completely modified to feed more people out or less acreage of land used, and this alteration has made this food dangerous to consume, now. The same parcel of land that used to produce a dozen loaves of bread now produces hundreds of loaves of bread. My question is how can the same land still pack as much nutrition in hundreds of loaves, as it did in a few dozen?

I contend that it can't. I contend that it's this mass production of this wheat, that's easier for the farmer, seed companies, and agrochemical companies to make a buck from, that's killing America and the rest of the world that consumes it. It may be giving pharmaceutical companies a booming business, but it's killing everyone who can't break the hold of its addiction.

What I've learned could fill volumes. To me, what's amazing is that I've retained a much greater portion of what I've learned, than I ever have in the past. This is solely due to the diet I've been on for the last 2½ years, 6 months in particular.

What makes me qualified to make the statements that I've declared in the book, is the fact that I've lived through it. I've been through the worst that this grain and food can put anyone through. Spending a month in a coma due to a drunk driver is about the worst expression that this addiction can do to anyone except kill them. In some cases, the latter of the two is preferential as the former leaves its victim with life changing injuries that are, most of the time, irreversible. I get to live with hemiplegia and it affects everything I do. Never-the-less, I kicked the addiction and I was addicted in the worst way.

My thinking is, if I can kick it anyone should be able to. But then I realize that there are million if not billions who are addicted worse than I ever was. This is evident in the obesity, diabetic, CVD, cancer and dementia epidemics that are so prevalent today. I also think, that if this diet can do this much to straighten me out, as bad as shape as I was in, to level out my emotions that have already been adjusted by a severe closed head injury, why couldn't it do the same thing for anyone else, who's brain damage may be different than mine, but never-the-less, still exists? Because of the nature of this food, everyone who's consumed it for any length of time, has brain damage.

Although their damage is quite different from mine, it's still brain damage and I know firsthand what brain damage does to a person. I know what severe brain damage does. I know what it's like to forget things. I know what it's like having trouble remembering things. I know what it's like to have mood changes that are completely out of character. Sounds a lot like Alzheimer's doesn't it? I can empathize with those losing their memories, as well as those who have to take care of them. I've been there. I've done that, more than once or twice or even three times. I'm well experienced at it.

That in itself, gives me the authority to state what I've stated throughout this book. Does one need a degree to see what this food is doing to us physically and well as what it's doing to our society? A little research was all I need to see the damage being inflicted on the American people. The studies aren't that hard to find. You just have to look for them. I just can't help but wonder, were these studies hidden on purpose? Did an industry, more interested in their bottom line, shade the reports of these studies, in an attempt to keep them stifled?

If an industry links itself with another industry that benefits each other, from the harm that one industry does, does that make them accomplices? We know how much the pharmaceutical industry takes from you for the treatment of all the disorders and diseases that this food inflicts upon you. Where would Bayer be without your headaches? Making crop seed? From what you've read here, in article 22 Bayer has already had in hands in both. So has Monsanto, Syngenta and a few others. This alarms me and it should you. This is a clear cut case, that what you don't know, is clearly killing you. To me, it's also the biggest ruse and crime ever committed on the American public. This is a change we must implement immediately if not sooner, but addiction keeps us from doing that.

I thought that was a good reason to write this book.

## WHY ARE THEY STILL PROMOTED LIKE THEY ARE?

## WHERE'S THE RECOMMENDATION FROM MORE DOCTORS TO STOP EATING THEM?

## WHERE'S THE RATIONALITY TO IT, EXCEPT FOR ADDICTION AND GREED?

# WHERE'S THE OUTRAGE?

# ABOUT THE AUTHOR

## **No one knows how hard it is for me to appear normal.**

### Living with hemiplegia.

At one time, I was just as I appeared to be, normal. But that was quite a while ago. Now it's a whole different story. Now, appearing normal is my biggest disability because nothing on the inside of me is as it appears on the outside. It takes more effort and energy than I can ever explain in one document just to appear normal. This statement, for example, I started it 30 minutes ago. I do the best I can and I don't hunt and peck type.

I took typing in the summer of my ninth grade and even though I never had the opportunity to use it, it stuck with me and came back a soon as I started typing again ten years ago. Even though I can type approximately 35 words a minute, I can't do it without errors. But those aren't the only errors that I encounter when I type out a document of this nature. In order for the document for portray an accurate account of my experiences, feelings, both physical and emotional, and actions, both wanted and unwanted, I constantly need to re-read it as I type it.

Even though my fingers are the most guilty parties, because of the multitude of times I *fat-finger* what I'm trying to type, they're not the main factor in my inability to finish this document in timely manner. The main factor is my inability to concentrate on what I'm writing about.

For that reason, I'll make a list of the problems that I get to deal with everyday and how they impact every aspect of my life that I can think of while I write this, knowing that there will be things that I will miss and need to update at a later time when I remember them.

- **Weakness on right side, all the time**
- **Slowness on right side, all the time**

- **Difficulty with balance, bowel control, vision in right eye, all of the time**
- **Trouble swallowing, hearing, holding on to things, most of the time**
- **Difficulty with memory, (mostly forgetfulness & short term memory) creating problems with understanding, reasoning, judgment, analyzing, deciding...etc, this happens every time I need to use these skills.**
- **Difficulty maintaining attention, keeping focused and intent to finish projects, and tasks. this happens whenever I need to concentrate on a task or project or focus on getting a job done. I call it neurological ADD.**
- **Think, speak, hear and read dyslexic, and I do it quite often**
- **Easily frustrated because of my inabilities often vocalizing my frustration at the top of my voice without control, hesitation or contemplation, too often**

All of these manifestations evolved after the severe closed head injury I sustained on December 24, 1984 as the result of a drunk driver running a red light and t-boning the car I was riding in. All of these problems are a direct result of the two bruises on my brain and strokes I sustained while comatose for 4 weeks due to that head injury.

For clarification purposes, I've now been working on this document for a little over 3 hours, to get this far and modified it again 5 hrs, later.

I will now try to explain how each of these manifestations affects the different parts of my life;

- **Weakness and slowness on right side**

I suffer from multiple problems all on the right side of my body. These problems include but are definitely not limited to: all the troubles and difficulties listed above, such as swallowing, hearing, vision, coordination, speed of movement, difficulty holding on to things – I'm always dropping things because I can't always feel my grip on them. I live with constant numbness (pins and needles) throughout my whole right side. My wrist always feels like it has a bunch of rubber bands around it that are always pulling and resisting every time I move a muscle. I never feel this on my left side. Every muscle on my right side has this *elastic* feeling.

My hip replacement is on the right hip probably because of my weakness on that side as well as my hernia, and chronic back ache in my lower back on right side. My right hand flops around every step I take, making it impossible to appear completely normal. Evidence of this can only be seen to an astute observer watching me walk. Whenever I take a step, my right hand flops around because of the lack of control I have over it. It's like my hand is held on my wrist by a bunch of rubber bands.

Because my right side is slower than my left, my right foot gets caught dragging behind, causing me to stumble. While just casually walking, it takes constant effort to walk without limping, due to the weakness on my right side. This is something that can be easily seen by everybody every time I run. I cannot run without a very noticeable limp. Even walking fast can't be done without a noticeable limp. I don't like walking fast or running because of the problems I've had in the past with balance, slow and weak right leg that won't work properly causing me to stumble or fall. I seldom walk anywhere without stumbling at least once because my right leg gets lazy and won't lift enough to clear the ground.

To avoid any of these problems, it takes an enormous amount of effort and energy. To appear normal, it takes even more effort and energy.

- **Trouble swallowing, hearing, holding on to things**

I often get food caught in my throat when several attempts to swallow it fail. I attribute that to the weakness on my right side no allowing my throat muscles to work as efficiently as the muscles on my left side where I didn't suffer any paralyses. I have the same problem holding on to things. Because I can't always feel what I'm holding in my right hand,

I often drop what I'm holding on to. Things seem to slip through my fingers more than they do with anybody else. Of the hearing problems I have, only hearing dyslexic is probably a result of the head injury. The tinnitus I have is probably due to the direct impact of the cars involved in the accidents that caused my injuries and the neck injury I received in another car accident in March of 1993. I say that the dyslexic hearing is a result of my head injury because of the trouble I have with my short term memory and not being able to recall the meaning of a particular word immediately. I often hear words spoken in reverse order because of this. I often speak my words in reverse order because of the same reason.

- **Difficulty with balance, bowel control, vision in right eye**

My balance is always questionable. Although I don't often lose my balance while on both feet, I can definitely balance on my left leg better than on my right leg. My right leg doesn't have the same amount of strength, endurance or ability to make the slight muscle changes necessary for balance, as my left leg has. That last reason alone is the major reason my balance problems persist.

The most embarrassing problem that I have to deal with, because it can sometimes be messy, is my ability to withhold a bowel movement. I attribute this to two factors; 1. That I'm not taking opioid medication anymore and enjoying a diet more rich in fruits and vegetables and 2. Weakness of my sphincter muscles to retain the fecal matter in my colon. Knowing that I always have at least two bowels movements each day, usually in the morning, I often have to stay close to a bathroom in the often case that I'll have to go a third or fourth time during the morning hours. I'm constantly making adjustments for this problem alone for there are times when I've had accidents while away from home.

Concerning the vision in my right eye, the clarity of the vision in my right eye grows weaker on its own, sometimes while I'm typing and can visually witness it and sometimes while I'm sleeping and wake up with diminished focus. Sometimes while I'm typing on my computer, I can remember when I realized a diminished focus in my right eye just recently. This wasn't the first time this has happened either. It's happened at least 3 times in the past 15 years. But it's only happened in my right eye.

- **Difficulty with memory, (mostly forgetfulness & short term memory) creating problems with understanding, reasoning, judgment, analyzing, deciding...etc, this happens every time I need to use these skills.**

This is quite often the most difficult disability to hide as it's always mistaken for stupidity or ignorance, when it's almost always a case or either poor judgment and poor decision making due to the inability of my brain to remember and think rationally and in a timely manner. When given time to organize my thoughts, I can prove to be very intelligent. Living without the ability to use this gift has proven to be a downfall for me. This is where my lack of short term memory has had the most effect on my life. Frustration hits me hard when I try to accomplish something I should be able to do in a specific amount of time, and can't. I either mess up the whole project, right at the finish of the project or can't even come close to finishing it in the time I should be able to. This often manifests itself in a very loud and very vulgar output that I have absolutely no control over. Anger issues are a common problem with head injuries of the nature I sustained and I think they're due exactly to this reason.

- **Difficulty maintaining attention, keeping focused and intent to finish projects, and tasks. this happens whenever I need to concentrate on a task or project or focus on getting a job done. I call it neurological ADD.**

This is caused by the same problems as my above problem with judgment and reasoning. When you can't remember what to focus on, how can you focus on anything? Lack of short term memory impacts a life more than almost anything else. You can never begin to understand what it does to interrupt a life until it happens to you and you have to live with it. These are *"shoes that not everybody gets to walk in"*, meaning only a few can fully understand the impact that no short term memory has on a life, and half of those that can, are are complete invalids. The other half are like me but you can usually see their disabilities. With me, you can't because of the trouble, effort and energy I put out to look like I'm not disabled. I'm not a complete invalid, just an unseen invalid.

- **Think, speak, hear and read dyslexic often**

I can't remember living with this problem before the head injury so I attribute this disability as well to my neurological damage. Quite often I'll say something dyslexic, or hear something dyslexic. Since my thinking is often dyslexic, I often type out my thoughts dyslexic as well. And this doesn't even come close to the number of times I read dyslexic. I see a lot of words and numbers backwards or letters within the word out of order. This always causes me to go back and re-read what I just read. I also have to re-read what I just read because I can't remember specific titles or names that I just read. You can only begin to fathom the problems that his can cause while I get to realize the full gamut of problems it actually does cause.

- **Easily frustrated because of my inabilities often vocalizing my frustration at the top of my voice without hesitation or contemplation**

This is the most damaging behavior caused directly by the neurological damage I sustained. Because of my recurring inabilities to complete projects and tasks, and verbalizing my frustrations in a vulgar manner, I'm always left feeling completely shamed from the action that I just presented, completely out of my control. I have no control over this behavior because all of my actions are actually reactions to my inability to complete or complete accurately, any project or task that I work on. It doesn't seem to matter how many times I say the serenity prayer, when frustration of my own inabilities decides to rear its ugly head, I have absolutely no control over how my brain is going to direct me to act. Again, you can only imagine the problems this kind of behavior can cause while I have to realize the full gamut of those problems.

I realize that the problems I experience are problems that a lot of other people experience, but how many people experience all of these problems on a daily basis, on an hourly basis or with the frequency that I do?

These are disabilities connected simply with the neurologic damage I live with, not the other disabilities I live with, in the form disabling pain in my back and groin and sometimes my hip. My back is sore when I get out of bed in the morning until I get back into bed at night, due to the degenerative disc disease and scoliosis I live with. The groin/testicular pain that I live with, comes on every afternoon, as I sit working at my desk. That pain has gotten severe enough to make me nauseous, at times. For twenty years, I've tried every known type of pain relief known to man, including opioid medication, nerve blocks, TENS, SCENAR, acupuncture, massage, topical balms, all without permanent success. The longest relief I've ever gotten, was from acupuncture. Most treatments lasted for a couple days, yet sometimes I had limited relief on the third day. This pain is the result of a hernia procedure that left what I was told is my genitofemoral nerve but I'd rather think it's my Ilioinguinal nerve because that's the nerve that branches out to the anterior scrotal nerve, trapped in scar tissue, which is where my pain emanates from.

The hip pain I experience is due to the hip replacement I had two years ago. I experience a stabbing pain, when I need to pivot on that hip, that almost takes my leg out from under me. I can walk up to ¼ mile painlessly. Thereafter the pain just keeps getting worse until I can sit or lay down.

My daily pain levels are as follows;

- Back pain – 2 when I wake up, 7 when I get out of bed with jabs to 8 or 9 following certain movements, 4 as I sit at my desk and work, 7 when I get up from my chair, 4-6 as I walk with right leg steps being very painful in the 8-9 range. When I go to bed at night the pain level as around the 4-6 range.
- Testicular/groin pain doesn't present itself until afternoon, depending on how long I need to sit at my desk. When it does it starts out in the 3-5 range increasing steadily in intensity for the rest of the day sometimes to the 8-10 range. (This is the pain that has made me suicidal.)
- Hip pain ranges from 0 when I wake up and get out of bed to 4-6 depending on how much I'm on my feet and walking. Twisting on that leg often provokes a stabbing pain jumping to 8 and often causes me to stumble.

I've now spent 4 hours on day 2 for this document to this point. I've updated it twice today after 3 times yesterday. I ended up spending about 8 hours on it yesterday.

I've had to live with this condition for the last 30 years, some of the pain for 40 years and some for only 20 years. I've searched for cures for my pain to no avail. I've even requested that my right testicle be removed, thinking that if there was nothing there to create the pain, the pain wouldn't exist, but was told time after time that I would have to live with phantom pain. So, I live with pain, sometimes massive pain, the kind that doubles you over.

This last edit took another 3 hours and includes 6-7 updates within the whole document. Even though I've updated this document 5 or 6 times, I'm still not sure I've listed everything necessary. Something keeps nagging at me that I just can't remember. All I can say is that when something affects every aspect of your life, as my neurological problems do mine, it's hard to cover everything in one document.

That was my last edit until I thought of some other things, while at church this morning that I should put in here. Now I just have to remember what they were...oh yes, the testicular pain that usually doesn't start until afternoon; that happens every day except Sundays when it hits me every Sunday in the morning while at church, from having to sit in a pew for an hours. Something else came to mind while in church this Morning, sure wish I could remember what it was...Oh yes, OCD, Obsessive Compulsive Disorder. Even though it hasn't been diagnosed, I think I do have a problem with it due to my ADD. Because I have to keep my mind occupied, I have this obsession with the game FreeCell. But then I had my obsessions before the head injury as well. They were just a little more difficult pursuits than what I'm capable of now, like bowling and golf and any other sport I was invited to play. Now, my obsessions are playing card games on the computer when I'm waiting on hold or any other time when I have nothing else to do. Thank God I do that when I'm alone. (FYI- last edit started over 6 hours ago, but I only spent about 5 hours typing and editing it. That's 6 days so far to complete this.)

**Addendum:** While not being able to understand any part of a paragraph I read, I re-read it two hours later with complete understanding. Every word that I didn't know before, my mind was able to recall when I read it the second time. My mind had 2 hours to work on the meaning of those words that I couldn't recall earlier without me even thinking about it. Not being able to recall the definitions as I was reading the paragraph, wouldn't allow me to understand it. But, I never would have understood it if I didn't re-read it, because I couldn't remember it.

**About the author** has not been edited due to the fact that I wanted to leave in the errors that were in the original document, so you could see the difference in my transformation.

www.ingramcontent.com/pod-product-compliance
Lightning Source LLC
Chambersburg PA
CBHW070231190526
45169CB00001B/154